KU-432-146

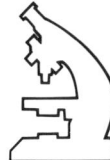

BASIC MICROBIOLOGY

EDITOR: J.F. WILKINSON

VOLUME 6

Plant Pathology and Plant Pathogens

C.H. DICKINSON

Department of Plant Biology
University of Newcastle-upon-Tyne

J.A. LUCAS

Department of Botany
University of Nottingham

SECOND EDITION

BLACKWELL SCIENTIFIC PUBLICATIONS

OXFORD LONDON

EDINBURGH BOSTON MELBOURNE

© 1977, 1982 by
Blackwell Scientific Publications
Editorial offices:
Osney Mead, Oxford, OX2 oEL
8 John Street, London, WC1N 2ES
9 Forrest Road, Edinburgh, EH1 2QH
52 Beacon Street, Boston
  Massachusetts 02108, USA
99 Barry Street, Carlton,
  Victoria 3053, Australia

All rights reserved. No part of this
publication may be reproduced, stored
in a retrieval system, or transmitted,
in any form or by any means,
electronic, mechanical, photocopying,
recording or otherwise
without the prior permission of
the copyright owner

First published 1977
Second edition 1982

Typeset by Santype International
Salisbury.
Printed and Bound by
Billings Book Plan,
Worcester.

DISTRIBUTORS

USA
  Blackwell Mosby Book Distributors
  11830 Westline Industrial Drive
  St Louis, Missouri 63141

Canada
  Blackwell Mosby Book Distributors
  120 Melford Drive, Scarborough
  Ontario, M1B 2X4

Australia
  Blackwell Scientific Book Distributors
  214 Berkeley Street, Carlton
  Victoria 3053

British Library
Cataloguing in Publication Data

Dickinson, C.H.
  Plant pathology and plant pathogens.—2nd ed.-
  (Basic microbiology; v. 6)
  1. Micro-organisms, Phytopathogenic
  I. Title   II. Lucas, J.A.   III. Series
  581.2′3   SB734

ISBN 0-632-00918-7

Contents

Preface to the second edition

The study of plant disease continues to be of paramount importance in maintaining and improving our food supplies. Although disease control remains the primary objective of pathologists the body of knowledge concerning other aspects of disease continues to increase dramatically. Our aim in this book is to provide a balanced treatment of all aspects of disease caused by microbial agents. Because disease caused by these agents is the end product of an interaction between a host and a micro-organism, emphasis is placed throughout on the host–pathogen complex. Wherever possible we have sought to develop general principles rather than give exhaustive lists of specific examples.

We have been given a great deal of encouragement and help in the preparation of this second edition. In particular we would like to thank J.A. Bailey, A. Bainbridge, I.R. Crute, C. Dickinson, J.T. Fletcher, M. Noble, M.J. Thresh and M. Wade for their helpful advice. S. Bell (and the Ministry of Agriculture Aerial Photography Unit), C.M. Brasier (and the Forestry Commission), M.D. Coffey, H.A.S. Epton, G.M. Farrell, J.T. Fletcher, R.T. Fox, J.T. Legg, J. Mansfield, K. Maramorosch, P.G. Markham, J.P. Ride, R.P. Scheffer, L. Seed, A.M. Skidmore (and ICI Plant Protection Division) and P.H. Williams have generously supplied us with photographic illustrations. A number of people deserve our thanks for their constructive criticisms of the new material incorporated in this second edition: A.O. Latunde-Dada, I.K. Knights and G. O'Hara. We would also like to record our appreciation of the invaluable material assistance rendered by B. Case, J.B. Green, V. Ross. R.H.T. Hall and P. Sanderson drew the diagrams to our complete satisfaction. Finally, Susan Dickinson and Bonnie Lucas deserve our thanks for their good humour during the revision of this book.

Colin H. Dickinson
John A. Lucas

Acknowledgments

Permission to reproduce data and figures from the following publications has kindly been given by authors, editors and publishers. References to this list are made at the appropriate point in the text.

AYRES P.G. & JONES P. (1975) *Physiol. Pl. Path.* **7**, 49.

BAILEY J.A. & DEVERALL B.J. (1971) *Physiol. Pl. Path.* **1**, 435.

BASHAM H.G. & BATEMAN D.F. (1975) *Phytopathology* **65**, 141.

BRACKER C.E. (1968) *Phytopathology* **58**, 12.

CAMPBELL W.P. & GRIFFITHS D.A. (1974) *Trans. Br. mycol. Soc.* **63**, 221.

CHRISTOU T. (1962) *Phytopathology* **52**, 381.

COFFEY M.D. (1975) *Symp. Soc. Exp. Biol.* **29**, 297.

COFFEY M.D. (1975) *Can. J. Bot.* **53**, 1285.

COFFEY M.D. (1976) *Can. J. Bot.* **54**, 1443.

CRAMER H.-H. (1967) *Plant Protection and World Crop Production.* Pflanzenschutz-Nachrichten, Bayer, 20.

DALY J.M., SEEVERS P.M. & LUDDEN P. (1970) *Phytopathology* **60**, 1648.

ECKERT J.W. (1977) In: *Antifungal Compounds*, Vol. I, *Discovery, Development and Uses*, p. 269. Marcel Dekker, New York.

ESAU K. (1968) *Viruses in Plant Hosts.* University of Wisconsin Press, Milwaukee.

EVANS E. (1977) In: *Systemic Fungicides*, p. 198. Longman, London.

FARRELL G.M., PREECE T.F. & WREN M.J. (1969) *Ann. appl. Biol.* **63**, 265.

FRY W.E. & THURSTON H.D. (1980) *BioScience* **30**, 665.

HARGREAVES J.A. MANSFIELD J.W. & ROSSALL S. (1977) *Physiol. Pl. Path.* **11**, 227.

HAYES J.D. & JOHNSTON T.D. (1971) In: *Diseases of Crop Plants*, p. 62. Macmillan, Basingstoke.

HEWITT H.G. & AYRES P.G. (1975) *Physiol. Pl. Path.* **7**, 127.

HICKEY E.L. & COFFEY M.D. (1977) *Can. J. Bot.* **55**, 2845.

HIRUMI H. & MARAMOROSCH K. (1973) *Ann. N. Y. Acad. Sci.* **225**, 201.

HOOKER W.J. (1956) *Am. Pot. J.* **33**, 47.

HOPPE H.H. & HEITEFUSS R. (1974) *Physiol. Pl. Path.* **4**, 25.

HULL R. (1974) In: *Biology in Pest and Disease Control*, p. 269. Blackwell Scientific Publications, Oxford.

JAMES W.C., SHIH C.S., HODGSON W.A. & CALLBECK L.C. (1972) *Phytopathology* **62**, 92.

JEFFREE C.E., BAKER E.A. & HOLLOWAY P.J. (1976) In: *Microbiology of Aerial Plant Surfaces*, p. 119. Academic Press, London.

KAARS SIJPESTEIJN A. & VAN DIJKMAN A. (1973) In: *Fungal Pathogenicity and the Plant's Response*, p. 437. Academic Press, London.

KRANTZ J. & ROYLE D.J. (1978) In: *Plant Disease Epidemiology*, p. 111. Blackwell Scientific Publications, Oxford.

KUĆ, J. (1971) In: *Microbial Toxins*, Vol. VIII, p. 211. Academic Press, New York & London.

LARGE E.C. (1952) *Pl. Path.* **1**, 109 [by permission of the Controller, HMSO].

LARGE E.C. (1954) *Pl. Path.* **3**, 129 [by permission of the Controller, HMSO].

LARGE E.C. & DOLING D.A. (1962) *Pl. Path.* **11**, 47 [by permission of the Controller, HMSO].

LIVNE A. (1964) *Plant Physiol.* **39**, 614.

LIVNE A. & DALY J.M. (1966) *Phytopathology* **56**, 170.

MAGYAROSI A.C., SCHÜRMANN P. & BUCHANAN B.B. (1976) *Plant Physiol.* **57**, 486.

MINAMIKAWA T. & URITANI I. (1964) *Arch. Biochem. Biophys.* **108**, 573.

MOORE W.F. (1970) *Pl. Dis. Rep.* **54**, 1104.

PITT D. (1976) *Trans. Br. mycol. Soc.* **66**, 239.

PRIESTLEY R.H. (1978) In: *Plant Disease Epidemiology* (eds Scott P.R. & Bainbridge A.), p. 63. Blackwell Scientific Publications, Oxford.

RIDE J.P. & PEARCE R.B. (1979) *Physiol. Pl. Path.* **15**, 79.

ROHRINGER R. & HEITEFUSS R. (1961) *Can. J. Bot.* **39**, 263.

ROYLE D. J. (1973) *Ann. appl. Biol.* **73**, 19.

ROYLE D. J. (1976) In: *Microbiology of Aerial Plant Surfaces*, p. 569. Academic Press, London.

SAMADDAR K.R. & SCHEFFER R.P. (1971) *Physiol. Pl. Path.* **1**, 319.

SCHEFFER R.P. & YODER O.C. (1972) In: *Phytotoxins in Plant Diseases*, p. 251. Academic Press, London.

SERMONTI G. (1969) *Genetics of Antibiotic-Producing Microorganisms*, p. 176. Wiley-Interscience, London.

STOVER R.H. (1973) In: *Crop Loss Assessment Methods*, FAO Manual on the Evaluation and Prevention of Losses by Pests, Diseases and Weeds. FAO and Commonwealth Agricultural Bureau.

THORNTON J.D. & COOKE R.C. (1974) *Physiol. Pl. Path.* **4**, 117.

TOMIYAMA K. (1971) In: *Morphological and Biochemical Events in Plant-Parasite Interaction*, p. 387. Denki Shoin, Tokyo.

WESTSTEIJN E. A. (1976) *Physiol. Pl. Path.* **8**, 63.

WILLIAMS P.H., AIST J.R. & BHATTACHARYA P.K. (1973) In: *Fungal Pathogenicity and the Plant's Response*, p. 141. Academic Press, London.

YOSHIKAWA M., YAMAUCHI K. & MASAGO H. (1978) *Physiol. Pl. Path.* **12**, 73.

1 Introduction

"We see our cattle fall and our plants wither without being able to render them assistance, lacking as we do understanding of their condition."
J. C. FABRICIUS (1745–1808)

Plant pathology is a science of synthesis. It draws upon data and techniques from fields as diverse as agriculture, microbiology, plant anatomy and soil science. In common with other broadly-based biological subjects, the evolution of ideas in pathology has become increasingly dependent upon advances in the fundamental areas of biochemistry and genetics. First and foremost, however, plant pathology is an applied science, involving practical solutions to the problem of plant disease. Part of the appeal of the subject as a field of study is to be found in this mixture of the pure and applied aspects of biology.

In the nineteenth century, following general acceptance of the germ theory of disease, great efforts were made to isolate and identify those micro-organisms responsible for particular diseases. An understanding of these causal organisms, and in particular of their life cycles and the ways in which they spread through a crop or survive under adverse environmental conditions, was seen as a prerequisite for devising adequate methods of control. This era of plant pathology was essentially one of description, and faced with the immediate problem of combating numerous destructive diseases, plant pathologists had little opportunity to explore fundamental aspects of host–pathogen interaction. Without such basic insights most of the early control methods were inevitably empirical, and many remain so even today.

The scope of plant pathology is difficult to define. Those who practise it are required to be conversant not only with the basic biological and agricultural sciences, but also with such apparently unrelated subjects as meteorology, aerodynamics, and even economics. On a practical level any shortcoming in the performance of a crop may be a problem for the pathologist. While theoretical pathology has moved towards a greater emphasis on diseases caused by microbial agents, in the field the pathologist is frequently faced with disorders caused by other factors. In this situation the pathologist may well be regarded in a similar light to the family doctor.

This might lead some to argue that field pathology is more of an art than a science!

An understanding of the biology of a single organism in isolation is only gained by intensive study. When the same organism is then considered in its natural habitat, subject to environmental fluctuations and competition from other organisms, its performance is even more difficult to assess. Consider then a host plant and a microbial pathogen separately in this way, and then combine the two. The result is surely one of the more complex situations the biologist has to unravel. The difficulties which must be faced in analysing a single disease are compounded by the diversity of host plants and the variety of agents capable of infecting them.

Due to the scale of these problems plant pathology has inevitably tended to fragment into separate specialized areas of study. For instance, insect pests are studied by entomologists, and mineral deficiencies by soil scientists. This book is primarily concerned with plant disease caused by micro-organisms. Many of the principles discussed apply equally well to disease caused by other agents. However, quite apart from the special place occupied by microbial pathogens in the history of the subject, the diseases they cause are of particular interest as they involve complex interactions between two living organisms. The relationships between green plants and their microbial parasites have also excited interest due to the varying degrees of evolutionary adaptation and specificity exhibited by these associations.

The interaction between a host and a pathogen involves four components (Fig. 1.1).

A comprehensive analysis of infectious disease must take all four components into account. Obviously one needs to be familiar with the characteristics of the host and the pathogen in isolation. The successful establishment of a pathogen in its host gives rise to a combination known as the host–pathogen complex. This is more than a simple sum of the two partners, as

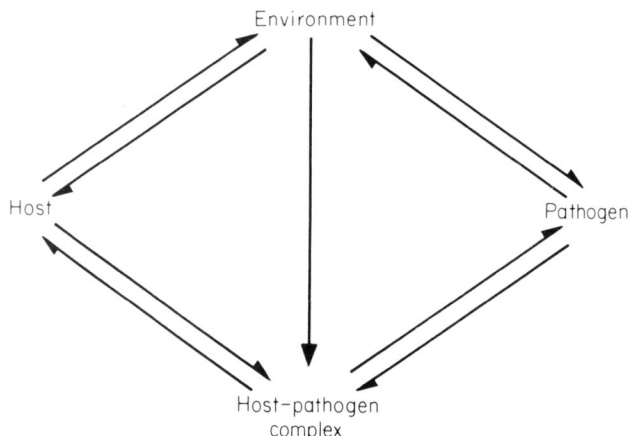

Figure 1.1 Host–pathogen interactions.

the properties of each are changed by the presence of the other. The effects of the environment on each of the other components must be known. In pathology, as in ecology, the environment includes not only physical and chemical factors but also macro- and microbiological agents. The two-way arrow between the host and the environment in Fig. 1.1 should not be overlooked, as populations of crop plants often have important effects on their surrounding microclimate. For example the relative humidity within a mature crop canopy is higher than that outside and this will favour the germination of spores. Effects of pathogens on the environment are more subtle but they can be significant; some fungi, for instance, produce the volatile hormone ethylene, which in turn affects the development of adjacent host plants.

This book is intended to provide a brief outline of the elements of modern plant pathology. The approach is designed to achieve a balance between laboratory and field aspects of the subject. The layout adopted follows the scheme outlined in Fig. 1.1. Separate consideration is given to the host and the pathogen. The host–pathogen complex is then considered as an entity in an account of the epidemiology of diseases caused by microorganisms. This account focuses on the environment as a major factor influencing the spread of pathogens. Later chapters deal with the host–pathogen complex in greater detail, first at the cellular and then at the molecular level; this leads on to a short discussion of the factors determining host–pathogen specificity, a subject of current interest due to its wider relevance to biological recognition systems. Finally, emphasis is placed on practical and applied aspects of the subject and the principles of crop protection are examined in the light of the earlier discussions.

A comprehensive treatment of individual diseases and the methods used in their control is obviously beyond the scope of a text of this length. For the sake of brevity, specific pathogens or the diseases they cause are often mentioned without further elaboration. This approach may be likened to that adopted in many ecology texts, in which the reader is expected to be familiar with the salient features of most of the higher plants or animals discussed therein. We have, however, included an appendix listing all the pathogens and diseases mentioned in the book, together with brief details which will enable the reader to acquire further information about particular disease syndromes. Further details of general aspects of pathology may be obtained by consulting the lists of recommended further reading.

FURTHER READING

General texts

AGRIOS G.N. (1978) *Plant Pathology*, 2nd edn. Academic Press, New York.
   A comprehensive and well-illustrated account of the subject with exhaustive coverage of all groups of pathogens
HORSFALL J.G. & COWLING E.B. eds (1977–80) *Plant Disease, An Advanced Treatise*, Volumes I–V. Academic Press, New York.
   A conceptual, rather than descriptive, approach with some especially interesting chapters.

WHEELER B.E.J. (1969) *An Introduction to Plant Disease.* John Wiley & Sons, London.
A systematic, crop-orientated description of disease.
See also the general texts listed on page 222.

Reviews and original articles

Many journals concerned with pure and applied research contain articles on, or relevant to, plant pathology. Amongst these, the following are especially useful:

Annals of Applied Biology
Canadian Journal of Plant Pathology
Netherlands Journal of Plant Pathology
Physiological Plant Pathology
Phytopathologische Zeitschrift
Phytopathology
Plant Disease
Plant Pathology
Transactions of the British Mycological Society

In addition, reviews of plant pathological topics can be found in the *Annual Review of Phytopathology*, *Biological Reviews* and *Review of Plant Pathology*.

2 The diseased plant

"It is of the first importance to understand that disease is a condition of abnormal physiology, and that the boundary lines between health and ill health are vague and difficult to define."
H. MARSHALL WARD (1854–1906)

At one extreme, disease in plants may be so severe that the need for preventative action or control measures is immediately obvious. The effects of specific pathogens or adverse environmental factors are apparent even to the casual observer. There are, however, many other diseases where it is difficult to define symptoms, where the cause of the problem is far from obvious and where any benefits obtained from control measures are not immediately apparent. In this chapter we will discuss what is meant by the term 'disease'. We will also survey the range of pathogens and environmental influences which adversely affect plants, and consider the significance of disease in agriculture and horticulture, where the economic consequences are the major concern.

CONCEPTS OF DISEASE

Plant pathologists seek to understand the nature and significance of disease. As a basis for this one must first identify the processes occurring during the growth and development of the healthy plant. Analysis of normal growth and development may be conducted at three different levels:
 (i) the sequence of events comprising a normal life cycle;
 (ii) the physiological processes involved in growth and development;
(iii) the molecular reactions underlying these processes.
   In many crop plants, seed germination, maturation of vegetative structures, the initiation of reproduction and the formation and dispersal of fruits and seeds are all critical phases at which disease may be manifested or assume special significance. At each stage in this developmental sequence, the integration of several physiological processes is essential for the continued development of the plant. Cell division and differentiation, the fixation and utilization of energy (photosynthesis and biosynthesis), transport of water and food materials (transpiration and translocation), and storage of reserve materials are all obvious necessities for growth. Each of these functions is related to a complex series of cellular and molecular events which

5

comprise the overall metabolism of the plant. The nature and direction of metabolism is itself an expression of the genetic make-up of the plant.

A logical extension of these considerations is that disease may disrupt the plant at one or more of the levels which we have identified. Some disorders involve subtle alterations in metabolism which do not affect the successful completion of the life cycle. Many diseases caused by viruses have only slight effects on the growth of the plant. In such cases it may be difficult even to recognize the existence of a disease problem. For instance, potato virus X was known as potato healthy virus until virus-free seed potatos became widely available. It was then shown to be capable of causing a 5–10% loss in yield. On the other hand, more destructive diseases may interfere with numerous molecular, cellular and physiological processes and lead to premature death of the plant.

Although we all have a fairly clear idea as to what disease is, in practice there may be difficulties in drawing a precise distinction between healthy and diseased plants. This is a problem that has been faced by many authors, as can be seen from the fact that no one definition has found universal acceptance in pathological texts. The most widely used definition of disease involves some reference to the 'normal' plant (see Further Reading—*Guide to the Use of Terms in Plant Pathology*). However, there is no consensus of opinion as to the exact extent of deviations from this norm which may constitute the diseased state. The problem of identifying normality, in terms of the processes outlined above, is further complicated by the variations inherent in all plant populations. Such variations are particularly common in natural populations, especially where hybrids occur, but even within apparently uniform populations of highly selected crop plants there may be considerable differences between individuals. Such differences either have a genetic basis or are due to environmental factors operating during the growth of the crop.

Damage or disease?

It can be argued that transitory deleterious effects on plants, such as injury due to grazing by cows or intermittent damage by lawn mowers, do not constitute disease! Indeed, some plants, such as the grasses, are especially well adapted to regular grazing and they respond with increased growth if so affected. In cases where damage is sustained over a longer period of time, e.g. progressive destruction of roots by herbivorous nematodes, or exposure to persistent herbicides, the outcome is clearly within the scope of pathology. However, these fine distinctions must be regarded as being of limited use in arriving at a working definition of disease. Such a definition will obviously depend in part on the situation in which it is intended to be used. For example, the biochemist may well be concerned with a malfunction involving a single enzyme and hence view disease as a specific metabolic lesion, whereas the farmer is normally only interested in changes

6

which reduce the value of his crop. In practice, plant pathology is concerned with disease identification and control, and economic considerations are obviously of overriding importance.

Although at present our definitions of disease lack precision, we may ultimately be able to describe all malfunctions on a precise biochemical basis. To date, this has been achieved in very few cases, for example, eye-spot disease of sugarcane caused by *Helminthosporium sacchari*, where all the symptoms may be attributed to the effects of a single toxin acting at a specific cellular site (see Chapter 8).

SYMPTOMS OF DISEASE

A doctor diagnoses illness in a patient by looking for visible or measurable signs that the body is not functioning normally. Such signs are known as disease SYMPTOMS and these may occur singly or in characteristic combinations and sequences. For example, someone suffering from influenza may have a sore throat, a high temperature and muscular aches and pains. Such a group of symptoms occurring together regularly is termed a disease SYNDROME. For many diseases the occurrence of a particular combination of symptoms is sufficient to arrive at an accurate diagnosis. Alternatively, symptoms may be common to a wide variety of diseases (for instance, fever is a generalized response to both infection and certain types of injury). If this is so, then detailed microbiological and biochemical analyses will be necessary to detect other diagnostic symptoms.

Similar considerations apply to the diagnosis of disease in plants. Just as with doctors and human disease, plant pathologists must be aware of the range of disease symptoms (Fig. 2.1) and what these suggest as the cause of the problem. The major symptoms of disease in plants are listed in Table 2.1 on the basis of the plant functions affected. This approach is useful because it directs attention to the underlying nature of the disorder. For instance, the presence of galls or other cancerous growths immediately suggests some malfunction in the control of cell division; this in turn implicates a hormonal imbalance and/or a genetic change in host cells. It should be realized that this classification of symptoms is to some extent arbitrary and non-specific. Permanent wilting provides a useful example. Although this symptom suggests that something is interfering with the uptake and transport of water, the symptom itself tells us little about the actual site or cause of the interference. The problem could be due either to a blockage in the vascular system, as in vascular wilt diseases, or to a general destruction of root tissues. It is also possible that the problem has nothing to do with water uptake or transport; in some diseases, e.g. potato blight, wilting is a sign of excessive water loss due to increased transpiration. The symptoms listed in Table 2.1 will interact in numerous ways. In club root of cabbage the basic symptoms are hypertrophy and hyperplasia in root tissue (Fig. 2.2), but the first visible symptom is often wilting of the aerial parts of the plant. Any disruption of normal root development inevitably affects other functions

7

such as water and nutrient transport. In view of the highly integrated nature of life processes, it is hardly surprising that attempts to categorize symptoms lack precision.

The relative importance of any symptom will vary, depending not only upon its duration and severity but also on the habit or life form of the plant affected (Table 2.2). Thus, necrosis in the stem of an herbaceous seedling

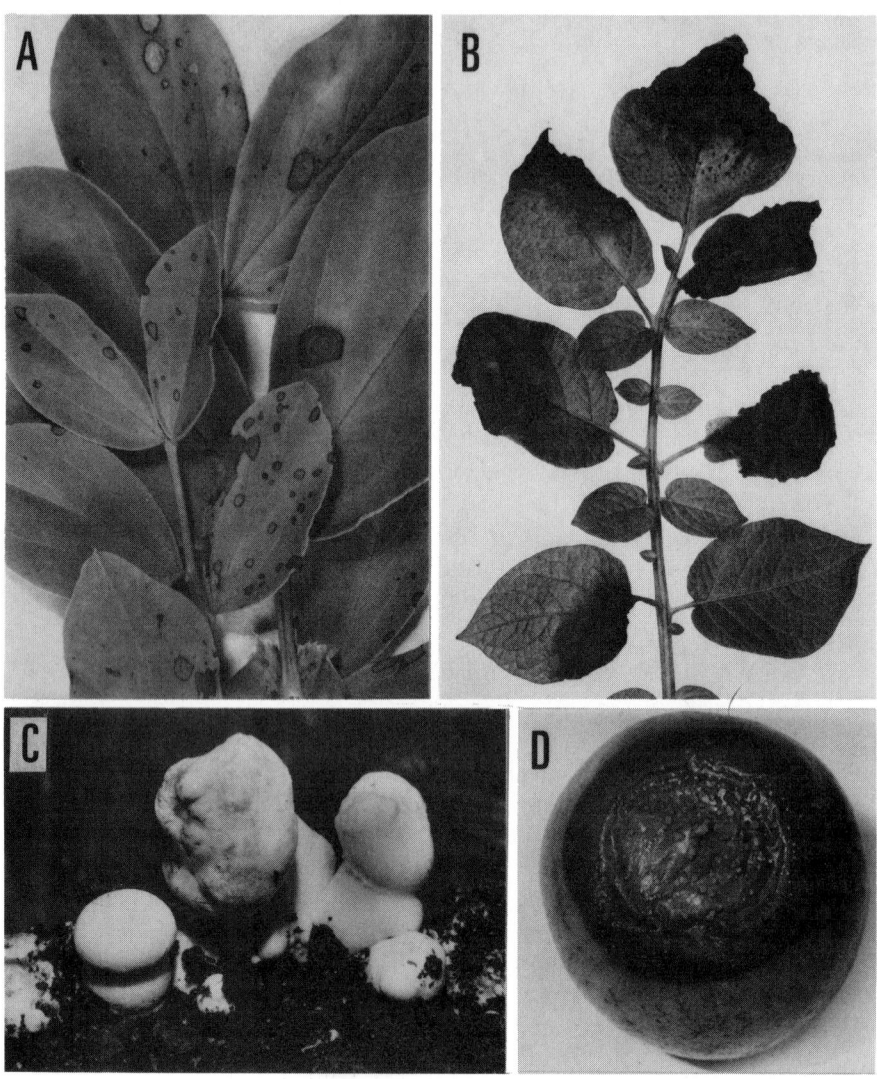

Figure 2.1 Plant disease symptoms. (A) Discrete, necrotic, chocolate spot lesions in broad bean leaves, caused by *Botrytis fabae*. (B) Extensive and rapidly spreading lesions in potato leaves due to the late blight pathogen, *Phytophthora infestans*. (C) Distorted fruit bodies of the cultivated mushroom. These symptoms are characteristic of dry bubble disease caused by *Verticillium fungicola*. (D) Brown rot symptoms on apple affected by *Penicillium expansum*. Concentric circles of fungal conidiophores indicate the position of the initial infection. (Photograph C by courtesy of J.T. Fletcher.)

Table 2.1 Symptoms of plant disease.

Symptom	Function affected	Examples
1. Necrosis (cell death)	General	Whole plant—Damping off Storage tissues—*Erwinia* soft rots of carrot and potato Leaf tissues—Potato blight Woody tissues—Apple canker, Fire blight
2. Chlorosis	Photosynthesis	Black stem rust, beet mild yellowing virus, aster yellows
3. Stunting	General development	*Pseudomonas* wilt of tobacco, barley yellow dwarf virus, apple rubbery wood
4. Permanent wilting	Water relations	Panama disease of bananas, *Verticillium* wilt of tomatoes, Dutch elm disease
5. Hypertrophy (abnormal cell enlargement)	Growth regulation	Club root of cabbage, white blister rust of crucifers, peach leaf curl
6. Hyperplasia (uncontrolled cell division)	Growth regulation	Crown gall, peach leaf curl
7. Leaf abscission	Growth regulation	Leaf cast of rubber, Gooseberry powdery mildew
8. Epinasty (downward growth of petioles)	Growth regulation	*Verticillium* wilt of tomatoes
9. Etiolation	Growth regulation	Bakanae disease of rice
10. Inhibition of flowering	Reproduction	Choke of grasses
11. Inhibition of fruit formation	Reproduction	Ergot on grasses, barley loose smut
12. Changes in pigmentation	Secondary metabolism	Peach leaf curl, tulip-breaking virus, grapevine leafroll virus

will probably lead to the death of the whole plant, but necrotic lesions in the stem of a woody perennial may result in nothing more serious than the loss of a twig or branch. If, however, such a lesion girdles the trunk of a tree, then translocation will be disrupted to the extent that the plant will die. Diseases which actually kill plants are the exception. More commonly, disease symptoms merely indicate an impairment of the efficiency of plant physiological and biochemical processes. Some symptoms, such as local changes in pigmentation, may be trivial in terms of overall plant performance. Often the most important consideration is the stage in the life cycle at which symptoms first appear. Severe chlorosis of the older, first-formed leaves of a cereal may have little effect upon the actual yield of grain, as most of the photosynthetic products required for grain filling are provided by the flag leaf and ear tissues. Accelerated abscission of leaves is unlikely to be a problem in annual herbaceous plants but in evergreen perennials it may exert a severe drain on the plants' food reserves. Such an effect can be seen in coffee trees affected by the rust fungus *Hemileia vastatrix* and in gooseberries affected with *Sphaerotheca* causing powdery mildew. In both instances early leaf fall is often followed by the production of a second crop of leaves. If these are also prematurely lost due to a second attack by the pathogen then the plant may die.

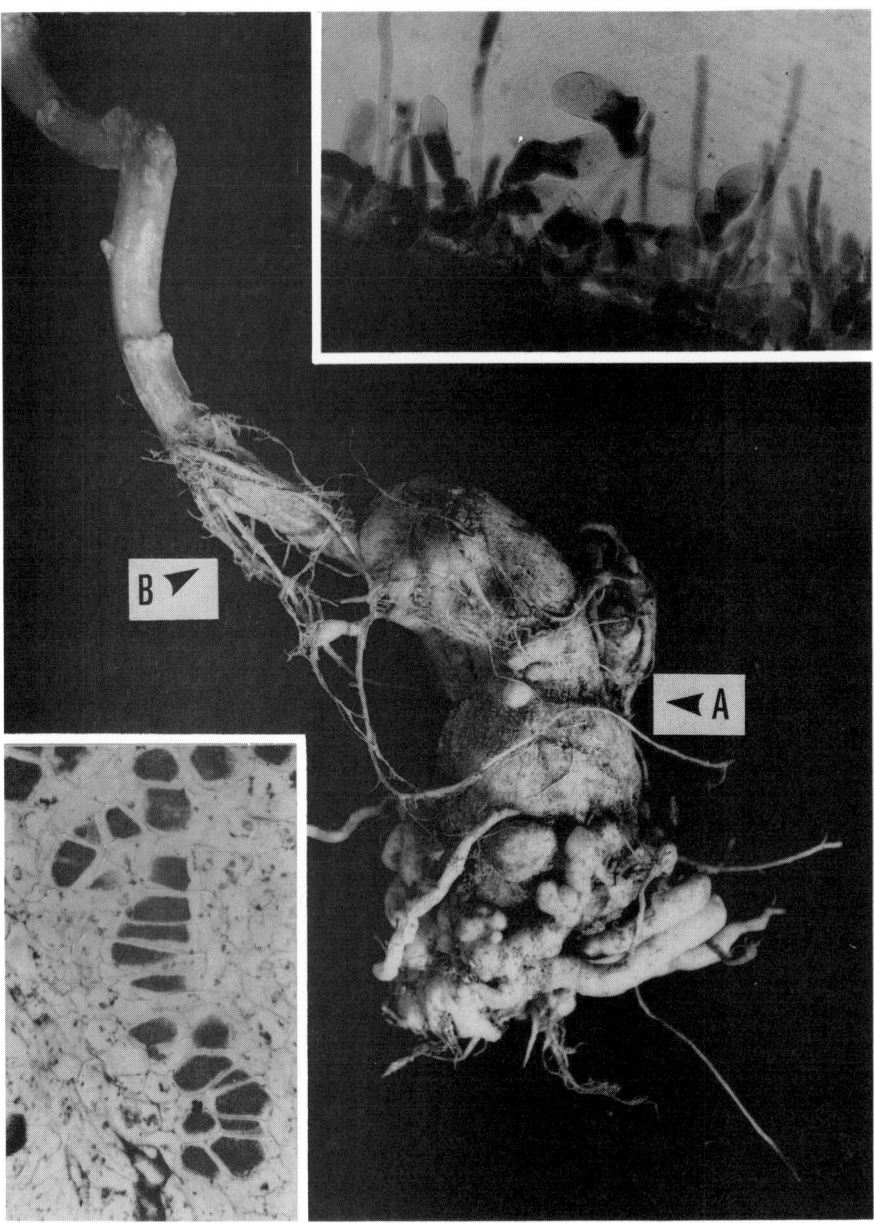

Figure 2.2 Club root disease of crucifers. Primary symptoms are seen in the inset picture at the top which shows distorted root hairs containing plasmodia of the fungal pathogen *Plasmodiophora brassicae*. Later the main roots become swollen (A) as compared with uninfected adventitious roots (B). These swellings are due to the repeated division and enlargement of the root's cortical cells, as is shown in the lower inset picture. (Main photograph by courtesy of ICI Plant Protection Division.)

Table 2.2 Symptoms in relation to function in higher plants.

| | Herbaceous Plants | | | | | Woody Plants | | |
| | Vegetative organs | | | Reproductive organs | | Vegetative organs | | |
	Roots	*Stems*	*Leaves*	*Flowers Fruit*	*Seeds Seedlings*	*Leaves*	*Stems*	*Roots*
Functions	Uptake Transport Anchorage	Support Transport	Photosynthesis Gas exchange Transpiration	Fertilization Development	Germination	Photosynthesis Gas exchange Transpiration	Support Transport	Uptake Transport Anchorage
Symptoms	Necrosis Hypertrophy Hyperplasia	Necrosis Etiolation	Hypertrophy Chlorosis Necrosis Epinasty Colour change Wilting	Inhibition Substitution Necrosis	Necrosis	Abscission Necrosis Wilting Chlorosis Hypertrophy Colour change	Necrosis	Necrosis
Disease examples	Root rots Club root	Foot rots Bakanae disease	Leaf spots and blight Leafroll Peach leaf curl Vascular wilts	Choke Ergot Anther smut Storage rots	Damping off	Coffee rust Leaf cast of rubber Panama disease of banana	Heart rots Cankers Fireblight	Root rots

CAUSES OF DISEASE

We define disease as a significant departure from normal metabolism and as such any agent capable of adversely affecting green plants may be regarded as lying within the scope of plant pathology. It would be tedious to assemble a comprehensive list of all the agents responsible for disease but the principal ones involved in the majority of diseases are listed in Fig. 2.3. Partial or total crop failure may be due to one or more factors. Where more than one agent is responsible, each may act independently or they may interact together. In the latter instance there may be SYNERGISM, that is, two or more agents acting in combination to produce changes which either is unable to produce in isolation.

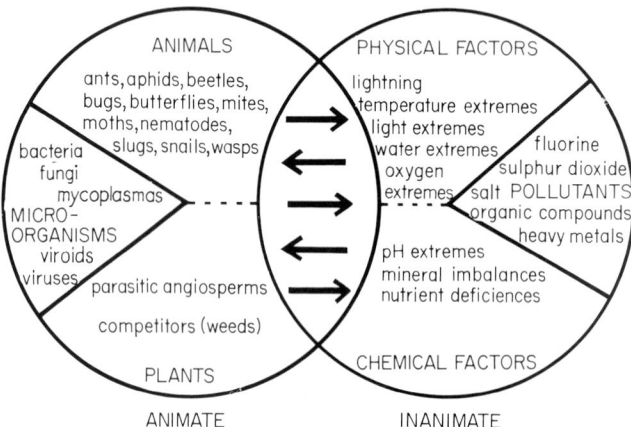

Figure 2.3   Agents responsible for plant disease.

Synergism has been demonstrated to occur with several combinations of viruses. For example, tobacco mosaic virus and potato virus X as separate infections cause relatively mild mottling symptoms in tomato. If by chance, however, they both occur together in the same plant then severe necrosis develops and this can even result in the death of the host.

A useful distinction can be drawn between animate and inanimate causes of disease (Fig. 2.3). Many of the animate agents, including the micro-organisms, the parasitic angiosperms and some of the animal pests, are infectious. Due to their capacity for growth, reproduction and dispersal, these agents spread from one host plant to another. Under particularly favourable circumstances, they may be dispersed rapidly over wide areas and even entire continents.

Pests

Amongst the animals attacking plants are many pests which cause only incidental damage to leaves, shoots, flowers, fruits and roots. Usually these pests, which include bark beetles, aphids, leaf hoppers and some nematodes, spend relatively brief periods on individual plants before moving on to explore new food supplies. Other pests, such as leaf miners, gall-forming sawflies and leaf-infesting nematodes, spend their entire life cycle or a major part of it on one plant. Animal attack may result simply in a drain on host nutrients or, alternatively, in extensive destruction of tissues. Aphids on leaves and stems extract sap from the phloem with an almost clinical efficiency. Many caterpillars are simply small herbivores; nevertheless they can consume large areas of the leaf lamina. Other animal pests cause more complex host responses or symptoms. Developing cynipid wasp larvae induce the formation of spectacular cherry or spangle galls on oak leaves, while certain nematodes cause swellings, termed 'knots', on the roots of tomatoes and potatoes. Such pests often show highly specialized adaptations to their respective hosts and, conversely, the plants are able to produce defence reactions in response to attack. These may be similar to those induced by micro-organisms which cause disease.

Parasitic plants

Higher plants may cause disorders of or damage to other plants, either by their adoption of a parasitic mode of nutrition or by acting as vigorous competitors or antagonists within mixed populations. Parasitic angiosperms are rare enough to be curiosities in many countries, but elsewhere they are nuisances or even serious, economically important parasites (Table 2.3). The dwarf misletoes can kill or deform pines and other conifers, and even minor attacks reduce the quality of timber by causing the production of numerous large knots and irregularly grained, spongy wood. Witchweed attaches itself to its host's roots by means of numerous haustoria. The parasite absorbs water and nutrients and this leads to wilting, chlorosis and stunting of the host.

Table 2.3 Angiosperms parasitic on other higher plants.

Family, common name, genus	Geographic area	Crops attacked
Convolvulaceae		
Dodder (*Cuscuta*)	Europe, North America	Alfalfa, clover, potatoes, sugar beet
Lauraceae		
Dodder (*Cassytha*)	Tropics and subtropics	Citrus trees
Loranthaceae		
Dwarf mistletoe (*Arceuthobium*)	Worldwide	Gymnosperms.
American true mistletoe		
(*Phoradendron*)	N. America	Angiosperm trees
European true mistletoe (*Viscum*)	Europe	Angiosperm trees, especially apple
Orobanchaceae		
Broomrape (*Orobanche*)	Europe	Tobacco, maize
Scrophulariaceae		
Witchweed (*Striga*)	Africa, Asia, Australia, N. America	Maize, sugarcane, rice, tobacco

The deleterious effects of other higher plants may, in contrast, be due merely to competition for space, light, water and nutrients. Species which are vigorous competitors with crop plants are usually described as WEEDS. In addition to these simple competitive effects, some plants produce chemicals which act in a manner similar to microbial antibiotics. The phenomenon whereby such chemicals inhibit the growth of neighbouring plants is known as ALLELOPATHY, but it is difficult to assess the extent to which this form of antibiosis operates in nature.

Inanimate agents

Green plants, in common with all other organisms, only flourish within a relatively narrow range of environmental conditions. Within the plant, individual cells are able to exert control over their internal environment and thereby maintain conditions suitable for normal metabolism. However, the extent to which living cells can withstand alterations in the external environment is limited. Fluctuations in environmental conditions outside an acceptable range are therefore harmful, and may result in irreversible damage to the plant. Green plants, unlike animals, are particularly susceptible to the effects of inanimate agents because they are sedentary and so are unable to escape from even local changes in the environment. Plants also lack the sophisticated homeostatic mechanisms possessed by higher animals.

Many inanimate disease agents are, under other circumstances, normal components of the environment. The harmful effects of physical factors are associated with the incidence of extreme values. For instance light, while essential for green plants, may in excess cause scorch diseases which result in the appearance of necrotic areas on susceptible aerial parts of the plant. Low temperatures often result in frost damage. Plants differ greatly in their sensitivity to frost and typical symptoms include morphological deformations or death of part or all of the plant. Many of these physical effects are relatively unsubtle and non-selective and the symptoms associated with them are non-specific.

In contrast, chemical deficiencies or imbalances often result in distinctive symptoms. These may be diagnostic in the case of deficiencies of essential cations. For example, magnesium deficiency in swedes is associated with an abnormal purplish pigmentation in interveinal leaf areas, whereas boron deficiency in the same crop causes brown-heart symptoms in the storage root. Deficiency diseases are commonplace, especially in the intensive cropping systems of present-day agriculture.

Excess amounts of certain mineral ions may be equally harmful, due to their effects on the availability or uptake of other essential ions. When insufficient iron is taken up, plants become chlorotic. Such a shortage may be due to inhibition of iron uptake by high levels of calcium or manganese in the soil, rather than to any absolute deficiency. Imbalances of soil nitrogen, phosphorus and potassium result in the development of plant tissues which are particularly prone to infection by micro-organisms or damage by other agents.

A common difficulty in diagnosing disorders caused by chemical agents is the similarity between the symptoms they produce and those due to infection by micro-organisms. Foliar symptoms in barley resulting from a deficiency of manganese resemble those caused by the leaf blotch fungus *Rhynchosporium*. Other deficiency diseases bear a striking resemblance to diseases caused by viruses.

Pollutants are substances which are either unnatural components of the environment, e.g. the polychlorinated biphenyls (PCB) and dichloro-diphenyltrichloroethane (DDT), or they are naturally occurring substances present in abnormal concentrations, e.g. fluorine, sulphur dioxide and sodium choride. Similarly high concentrations of some pollutants may be a normal feature of other habitats, but problems arise when man redistributes these substances. Salt concentrations which are non-toxic to salt marsh plants severely injure inland species exposed to roadside salt splash following de-icing.

The influence of many of these compounds on higher plants is now well known and the symptoms induced include abnormal growth due to meristem damage, chlorosis and necrosis. Some species of plants are especially sensitive to particular pollutants. However, within a species the response of different cultivars to a compound may vary considerably. These variations are essentially similar to variations in the response of different cultivars to microbial attack.

In this discussion, we have only considered the direct effects of biological, physical and chemical agents acting independently. In reality, all these agents interact with each other in a more or less complex manner. For instance, high light intensity is accompanied by an increase in temperature. This increase in itself will have further effects in accelerating water loss. It is difficult, therefore, to distinguish between the damaging effects of each of these factors. Other interactions are even more complex. Relatively low concentrations of sulphur dioxide are toxic to many plants, but traces of this gas are even more toxic to fungi. As a result some fungal diseases, such as black spot of roses (caused by *Diplocarpon rosae*), are unknown in polluted cities or other industrialized areas, although their potential hosts are still able to thrive.

SIGNIFICANCE OF DISEASE

Disease is commonplace in most agricultural crops. In the majority of outbreaks, however, little effort is made to do more than either minimize the losses caused or compensate for expected shortfalls in yield by overplanting. The ideal situation in which pathogens are avoided, excluded or totally eliminated is the ultimate goal for students of plant pathology; practising plant pathologists and agriculturalists usually compromise in aiming to limit disease to acceptable levels.

In natural communities, disease is just one of the many factors which regulate populations and hence determine the spectrum of species which are successful in any habitat. In particular, disease will tend to limit the spread of species to less favourable geographic regions or habitats, as many pathogens are more virulent when their hosts are growing under suboptimal conditions. Disease may also accelerate change within established plant communities. For example, forest trees may be killed, thereby opening the canopy and allowing regeneration to proceed.

One of the problems in discussing the significance of disease is that there is no universally accepted scale by which it is rated. This is partly because there are so many different types of disease which affect agricultural production; it is also a consequence of the diverse interests of the various people involved in crop husbandry. Farmers and foresters are, by and large, interested only in those changes in crop performance which influence quantitative and qualitative aspects of yield, and hence their cash return per hectare. For many years, farmers tended to regard disease in rather the same way as they view the weather–something to consider philosophically as a natural hazard but rarely to do anything about! To a certain extent this is still true today in that any preventative measure that is available will be thought of in terms of financial expediency. Even a possible bonus, such as restricted carry-over of the disease agent until the following season, may not provide sufficient incentive for any financial outlay.

Other parties interested in plant diseases are Government advisory or extension pathologists and the chemical industry. Advertising pressure is exerted on farmers by the chemical industry, seeking to promote the sales of agrochemicals. Government pathologists assess the comparative performances of commercial formulations under field conditions, enabling them to make recommendations as to the relative efficacy of certain chemicals. These pathologists also evaluate the possible advantages of chemical or biological control measures. However, in most instances, they are unable to predict precisely the future development of the disease, and their advice, which may involve the expenditure of time and money, can only be a matter of judgement. For these reasons the approach adopted is usually relatively conservative.

The relationship between the chemical industry and research pathologists is not entirely satisfactory, as the availability of information concerning the activity, formulation and environmental side-effects of the products is often restricted. However, following demonstration of the deleterious environmental effects of some pesticides, pressure has been applied, both through legislation and voluntary schemes, for more stringent assessment of the toxicity of new compounds. This has inevitably created extra difficulties in the development and registration of new agrochemicals and so has added to the costs incurred prior to market release (see also Chapter 10).

The relationship between the amount of disease and loss of income is complex. A theoretical analysis of this relationship is outlined in Fig. 2.4.

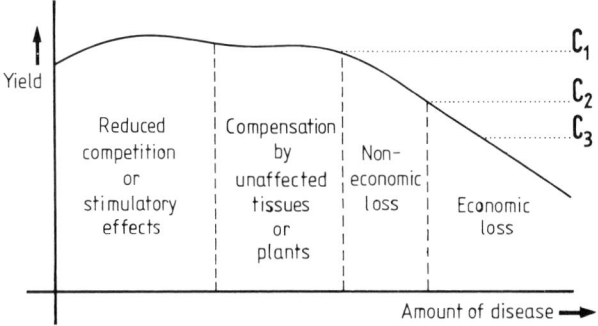

Figure 2.4 Theoretical relationship between amount of disease and yield. Yield reduction $(C_1 - C_2)$ approximates to the acceptable shortfall in the performance or harvesting of the crop. Below C_2 crop income is reduced, but control measures are not justified until $C_2 - C_3$ is greater than the cost of the treatment.

Difficulties arise in the practical application of such models due to the many possible interactions between symptoms of disease and the final determinants of crop yield.

The impact of disease

In the foregoing discussion we have deliberately minimized the significance of disease, as we are of the opinion that all too frequently the impression is given that the battle against pathogens is always being waged at full pitch. This is not so and although disease takes a steady toll from all major crops (Table 2.4), only occasionally are losses severe enough to be a matter of life and death. One can, however, cite many cases where the impact of plant disease has been such that the course of history has been changed. No one would seek to underestimate the tragic effects of potato blight in Ireland during the 1840s or the devastation wrought by coffee rust in Sri Lanka in the late nineteenth century. Recently, coffee rust has spread to South

Table 2.4 Estimated annual world losses, in tonnes $\times 10^6$, due to diseases, pests and weeds (data from Cramer, 1967*).

Commodity	Potential production	Losses due to Diseases	Insect pests	Weeds	Actual production
Wheat	356.8	33.8	18.1	35.1	269.8
Rice	445.7	40.0	122.6	47.4	235.7
Maize	344.9	33.2	44.7	45.0	222.0
Potatoes	406.4	90.3	24.2	16.8	275.1
Sugar (beet and cane)	1351.7	236.0	232.1	177.9	705.7
Vegetables	284.4	31.6	23.8	24.1	204.9
Fruit	200.4	33.1	11.5	11.8	144.0

* Full references for data and figures acknowledged in the text are given on pp. vii–viii.

America with serious consequences for the economies of many of the world's major coffee producers. Diseases such as these have taken a dreadful toll in terms of human suffering. Other diseases, including white pine blister rust, chestnut blight and downy mildew of grape vines, have precipitated major changes in agriculture or natural landscapes over vast areas. Nor are such devastating disease epidemics a thing of the past. The major epidemic of Southern corn leaf blight in the United States in 1970 has raised doubts about the wisdom of achieving genetic uniformity in modern cereal crops and forced a reassessment of the breeding methods employed in the production of new cultivars.

Even in areas of high agricultural efficiency, disease losses may make highly significant inroads into profits (Table 2.5). Although it would be

Table 2.5   Cereal yield losses in England and Wales, 1972–1980, caused by foliar pathogens. Losses are based on mean yields (4.8 tonne/ha for spring barley and 5.2 tonne/ha for winter wheat) and 1981 prices (£92 and £105 per tonne for barley and wheat respectively). (Data from Agricultural Development and Advisory Service, UK.)

| | LOSSES (M£) | |
	Spring barley	Winter wheat
1972	81.2	63.0
1973	139.5	51.6
1974	74.7	25.2
1975	60.6	18.6
1976	71.2	12.8
1977	41.2	13.9
1978	60.7	34.4
1979	40.2	35.4
1980	62.3	20.4

presumptuous to argue that modern agriculture is especially prone to disease outbreaks, the astronomic and continuing increase in world population, with all its attendant pressures on agriculture, would seem to have increased our vulnerability. The need for improved agricultural productivity has led to vast areas being planted with high-yield, genetically identical cultivars. Similarly, the increasing cost of labour and the trend towards mechanization, which involves large-scale capital expenditure, have also contributed to a reduction in the range of crop types planted. As a result, long-hallowed principles of crop rotation have been abandoned in some areas.

A second aspect of modern agriculture which has undoubtedly aggravated disease problems is increased world trade in crop plants and plant products. Following the gradual shift from self-sufficiency, at a community and in many instances also at a national level, large-scale transport of plant material and food produce has become commonplace. The consequences of such transportation over long distances are well known. One need only cite the introduction of Dutch elm disease into North America in the 1930s, and the recent re-introduction of a virulent strain into the U.K. on imported elm logs, to emphasize the hazards of exposing host plants to foreign races of the pathogen. In addition, there is an increasing need for long-term storage of produce, which, in its turn, brings further pathological problems. Losses due to post-harvest diseases have tended to be underrated. In actual fact, with some crops, spoilage while in store is the single most important source of loss. It has recently been estimated that one third of all tropical produce is destroyed, by a variety of agents, before it reaches the consumer. Even in highly developed countries, the scale of potential losses during the long-term storage, transport and marketing can be daunting (Table 2.6). The recognition that such losses occur regularly has provided a powerful incen-

Table 2.6 Estimates of post-harvest losses likely to occur in the absence of effective disease-control measures (data from Eckert, 1977).

	Commodity	Country of origin	Potential loss %
Loss during low-temperature storage	Apples	England, USA	2–50
	Carrots	England, USA	6–38
	Citrus fruits	Italy, USA	3–52
Loss during transport and marketing	Apples	USA	29
	Citrus fruits	USA	0–25
	Lettuce	USA	10–15
	Peaches	USA	15–24
	Strawberries	USA	25–35

tive for the development of pesticides specifically designed to protect the crop in store and has emphasized the value of rapid-processing systems, such as canning and freezing, which prevent any post-harvest microbial spoilage.

All in all, the intensification of agriculture through plant breeding, by the manipulation of the environment and by the widespread use of chemical growth regulators has brought in its wake new and sometimes severe disease problems. While it is true that breeding programmes and chemical control measures have won notable victories in the war against plant disease, it should be realized that the innovations which at first sight appear beneficial can backfire. Irrigation has opened up whole new regions to agriculture, but the same water which brings life to the crop can also nourish and spread its microbial enemies.

FURTHER READING

General texts

AINSWORTH G.C. (1981) *An Introduction to the History of Plant Pathology.* Cambridge University Press, Cambridge.
A carefully documented and detailed description of the development of the science of plant pathology.

Buczacki S. & Harris K. (1981) *Guide to the Pests, Diseases and Disorders of Garden Plants.* Collins, London.

A practical, well-illustrated, descriptive account of disease, with strong emphasis on the use of symptoms to identify problems.

Gunn D.L. & Stevens J.G.R. eds (1976) *Pesticides and Human Welfare.* Oxford University Press, Oxford.

A broad statement of the problem with an ecological slant, sponsored by the agrochemical industry.

Ordish G. (1976) *The Constant Pest.* Peter Davies, London.

A thoroughly readable account with an historical bias.

Reviews

A Guide to the Use of Terms in Plant Pathology. *Phytopathological Papers,* No. 17. Commonwealth Mycological Institute, Kew, England.

Crowdy S.H. & Manners J.G. (1971) Microbial disease and plant productivity. *Symposium of the Society of General Microbiology* **21**, 103–123.

Klinkowski M. (1970) Catastrophic plant diseases. *Annual Review of Phytopathology* **8**, 37–60.

Thurston H.D. (1973) Threatening plant diseases. *Annual Review of Phytopathology* **11**, 27–52.

3 The microbial pathogens

"It was first necessary to determine if characteristic elements occurred in diseased parts of the body, which do not belong to the characteristics of the body, and which have not arisen from body characteristics."
ROBERT KOCH (1843–1910)

Heterotrophic organisms, unlike autotrophs, are entirely dependent upon an external supply of organic carbon compounds. The ultimate source of most carbon compounds is green plants. There are, however, a variety of routes by which microbes can obtain these compounds from green plants.

A large number of micro-organisms are decomposers. These organisms utilize substrates in dead or moribund tissues and their activities eventually lead to the disappearance of plant and animal remains. Some decomposers have, in addition, an ability to attack living plants; if, as often happens, they kill the plant, this ensures a supply of moribund tissues on which they can continue to grow. Other micro-organisms are only able to obtain nutrients from living host plants. The effects that these organisms have on their hosts range from very limited disruption of normal functions to drastic damage which may even threaten the life of the plant. It can be seen, therefore, that heterotrophic micro-organisms are involved in a variety of ways in the movement of fixed carbon between different trophic levels in ecosystems. They thus play a key role in the carbon cycle (see *Microbial Ecology*, Volume 5 in the Basic Microbiology series).

The identification of microbes responsible for plant disease implies two steps. In the first place organisms must be considered in terms of the methods they use to obtain nutrients from living and/or dead plants. Secondly, they must be identified taxonomically. However, the usual taxonomic criteria employed in identifying microbial species may be of limited value when dealing with micro-organisms isolated from their host plants. Many of the characteristics of major significance in pathogenesis are subject to considerable intraspecific variation. For example, the damage inflicted on a host by different isolates of the same species can vary considerably. Analysis of the genetic basis of this variation, which involves corresponding variations in the host's response, is a further necessary step in understanding infectious disease.

PATHOGENS AND PATHOGENESIS

A great deal of confusion surrounds the terms pathogen and parasite. While they are generally reserved for description of microbial disease agents, in particular, the fungi, bacteria and viruses, the distinction between the two words has often been overlooked. They are not synonymous; a parasite is an organism having a particular type of nutritional relationship, while the term pathogen refers to the ability of an organism to cause disease. They may be defined as follows.

PARASITE: an organism or virus existing in intimate association with another living organism (host) from which it derives some or all of its nutrients, while conferring no benefit in return.

PATHOGEN: an organism or virus able to cause disease in a particular host.

The allied term PATHOGENESIS describes the complete process of causing a disease, the sequence of events from initial infection to production of symptoms.

At first sight the distinction between a parasite and a pathogen might appear relatively minor; indeed in many cases the parasitic activities of an organism automatically lead to it being a pathogen as well. The diversion of nutrients from the host will inevitably lead to some metabolic stress which will normally be expressed as disease. However, in other host–microorganism associations this stress may be offset by the microbe contributing or being deprived of other nutrients in return. This is the case with root nodules of legumes, where the bacterium *Rhizobium* obtains carbohydrates from the host but also fixes atmospheric nitrogen which the host subsequently utilizes. The definition of a parasite given above takes account of situations such as these.

Where the invading microbe confers some beneficial effect the term SYMBIOSIS has been used. As originally conceived, however, symbiosis referred to any intimate or close association between two organisms, irrespective of their effects on each other. Thus symbiosis includes both antagonistic (i.e. parasitic) and mutually beneficial associations. The term MUTUALISM is now preferred for the latter type of association. The major types of mutualistic association involving plants and micro-organisms are listed in Table 3.1.

If one considers the terms parasite and pathogen from the reverse viewpoint, in other words the ability to cause disease, the difference becomes more obvious. While all parasites are to some extent pathogenic due to their redirection of host nutrients, many of the characteristic symptoms of disease cannot be explained on the basis of nutritional stress alone. The growth and development of a pathogen in its host, along with the response of the host to the presence of an alien organism, involves other interactions which have little to do with nutrition. Many of the more injurious effects of pathogens may be traced to chemical factors whose production is apparently incidental to their parasitic way of life (see Chapter

Table 3.1 Mutualistic associations between higher plants and micro-organisms.

	Partners involved and their contribution to the association	
Lichens	Green algae Cyanobacteria Organic carbon, plus organic nitrogen from cyanobacteria	Fungi (mainly Ascomycotina) Water and inorganic nutrients
Seedlings Orchidaceous mycorrhizas	Orchids Contribution not known	Fungi (e.g. *Rhizoctonia* species) Simple carbohydrates and inorganic nutrients
Stems Stem nodules	*Gunnera* Basic requirements for growth	*Nostoc* Fixed nitrogen
Leaves Leaf nodules	Rubiaceae and Myrsinaceae Basic requirements for growth	Bacteria Growth factors
Roots Arbuscular mycorrhizas	Angiosperms Contribution not known	Fungi (Endogonaceae) Inorganic nutrients especially phosphorus
Ectomycorrhizas	Broadleaved trees and conifers Carbohydrates	Fungi (Basidiomycotina) Inorganic nutrients
Root nodules	Legumes *Alnus* Basic requirements for growth	*Rhizobium* *Frankia* (actinomycete) Fixed nitrogen

8). Looked at in this way, the statement 'a good parasite is a poor pathogen' has some meaning. Any organism which is dependent upon another organism for its supply of nutrients might be expected to restrict its pathogenic effects to a minimum.

Biotrophs and necrotrophs

Although there is an enormous variety of pathogens, an important distinction can be made between those which rapidly kill all or part of their host, and others which coexist with host tissues for an extended period without inflicting severe damage. The former category, referred to as NECROTROPHS, are often opportunist pathogens which invade wounds and juvenile or debilitated plant tissues. They grow intercellularly producing cytolytic factors and then utilize the dead host tissues as a substrate. The ability to attack a living host distinguishes these organisms from the obligate SAPROTROPHS which subsist exclusively on organic debris.

In contrast, BIOTROPHS do not kill their host immediately. They are, in fact, dependent upon viable host tissue to complete their development. At its most extreme, biotrophy approaches mutualism in that it may be difficult to discern any marked pathogenic effects. The contrasting features of necrotrophs and biotrophs are summarized in Table 3.2.

Biotrophs, in keeping with their more specialized form of parasitism, attack only a limited range of hosts. Biotrophic fungi frequently form intra-

Table 3.2 Major characteristics of necrotrophic and biotrophic pathogens.

Necrotrophs	Biotrophs
Biochemical and morphological features	
Host cells rapidly killed	Host cells not rapidly killed
Toxins and cytolytic enzymes produced	Few or no toxins or cytolytic enzymes produce[d]
No special parasitic structures formed	Special parasitic structures, e.g. haustoria, typically formed
Host penetration via wounds or natural openings	Host penetration direct or via natural opening[s]
Ecological features	
Wide host range	Narrow host range
Able to grow saprophytically away from the host	Unable to grow away from the host
Attack juvenile, debilitated or senescing tissues	Attack healthy hosts at all stages of developme[nt]

cellular feeding structures which are termed haustoria (see Chapter 7). Generally speaking, these fungi do not produce large quantities of extracellular enzymes or toxins; during their coevolution with the host, synthesis of degradative enzymes may have been repressed, and their ability to elaborate such enzymes eventually lost altogether (see Lewis, 1973). An alternative view of the relationship between necrotrophs and biotrophs is that the former have evolved from the latter through an increasing ability to produce enzymes capable of degrading complex substrates (see Cooke & Whipps, 1980). The impression may have been given that biotrophy and necrotrophy represent absolute categories. However, as is the case with all man's efforts to compartmentalize nature, there is in reality a continuous gradation between the two types of pathogen. At one extreme are the viruses, which require a living cell within which to reproduce, and fungal biotrophs, such as the downy and powdery mildews. At the other extreme are typical necrotrophs, such as the damping-off fungi and soft-rot bacteria. In between, one encounters pathogens with intermediate characteristics. For instance, *Phytophthora infestans*, the potato late blight fungus, exhibits a high degree of host specificity and other biotrophic features such as haustoria, but it also causes relatively rapid necrosis of invaded tissues. Some pathogens pass through both a biotrophic and a necrotrophic phase during their life cycle. The apple scab fungus, *Venturia inaequalis*, grows beneath the cuticle of host leaves for several weeks without causing obvious necrosis but as the lesions age, host tissues are eventually killed and the typical scabs develop (see Fig. 10.2).

Evolutionary speculations as to the origin of parasitism have tended to support the idea that necrotrophs are more primitive parasites than biotrophs. In the absence of any useful fossil record this conclusion is based on the assumption that evolutionary advances are accompanied by increased specialization. It is possible, however, that secondary simplification of certain features has occurred. At first sight such simplifications might suggest that an organism is relatively primitive. Morphologically, the viruses appear to be primitive but in all other respects they may be regarded as the ultimate biotrophic parasites in terms of the subtlety of their interactions with the host at the subcellular level.

In nature, necrotrophs may grow on both living and dead host tissues. Pathogens such as *Pythium* and *Rhizoctonia* may be found growing actively in soil, or on subterranean or aerial plant surfaces in competition with the natural microflora. Even in the absence of a suitable host they may successfully complete their life cycle by utilizing dead organic substrates. The ability of biotrophs to compete with other micro-organisms for dead organic matter is very limited or even non-existent. These differences in patterns of natural occurrence of pathogens are reflected in their growth on laboratory culture media. Most necrotrophs are nutritionally undemanding; they grow satisfactorily on a wide range of relatively simple media and may compete successfully with obligate saprotrophs for organic debris. Biotrophs, on the other hand, have traditionally been regarded as nutritionally exacting organisms and in extreme cases individual species or groups cannot be grown on any known culture media. Distinctions based on the criterion of culturability have been, and still are, used to divide pathogens into two nutritional types, FACULTATIVE and OBLIGATE parasites. A further refinement of this scheme distinguishes pathogens which are able to grow relatively well in pure culture, but which in nature are unable to compete with non-parasitic microbes in the surrounding environment. Such pathogens are termed ECOLOGICALLY OBLIGATE in contrast to BIOCHEMICALLY OBLIGATE organisms which are unable to grow apart from the living host either *in vivo* or *in vitro*. This latter group are presumed to have special nutritional or other requirements which are provided only by living host tissue.

However, in recent years it has been discovered that certain fungi which were once thought to be nutritionally demanding can be cultured on relatively simple media. This has blurred the distinction between facultative and obligate parasites. Several species of rust fungi, originally regarded as strictly obligate parasites, have now been successfully cultured away from their hosts. While there is still some controversy as to whether these cultures represent mutant strains which bear little resemblance to wild types, the criterion of culturability has, nevertheless, lost much of its usefulness.

In taxonomic terms the delimitation of species of pathogenic micro-organisms is based on the usual morphological and physiological criteria. However, many of the taxa thus created are inadequate for identification of pathogenic isolates of fungi and bacteria. Isolates which appear identical according to conventional criteria show physiological specialization on particular host species; yet this character is not recognized in the classical taxonomic approach. In instances where this specialization is clear cut, it may therefore be possible to recognize FORM SPECIES of fungi. For instance, the black stem rust fungus occurs as a number of form species, including *Puccinia graminis* f.sp. *tritici* on wheat and *P. graminis* f.sp. *hordei* on barley. A corresponding scheme has been suggested for bacteria, where the term pathovar may be used to accommodate isolates with an ability to cause disease in specific groups of host plants.

KOCH'S POSTULATES

Amongst the syndrome of symptoms which is the hallmark of a particular disease one often sees a micro-organism which is presumed to be the pathogen. To determine with certainty that this micro-organism is the cause of the disease rather than some incidental contaminant it is necessary to examine critically its relationship with the host plant. This dilemma was first recognized in studies on microbial pathogens of man. In 1876, Robert Koch provided the first experimental proof of disease causation by applying a set of rules which have since come to be known as Koch's postulates. Koch considered that these rules must be satisfied before any micro-organism can be regarded as a pathogen. The rules may be summarized as involving five step-wise operations, outlined below.

1   The suspected pathogen must be consistently associated with the same symptoms.
2   The organism should be isolated into culture, away from the host. This precludes the possibility that the disease may be due to malignant tissues or other disorders of the host itself.
3   The organism should then be re-inoculated into a healthy host.
4   Symptoms should then develop which are identical to those observed in the original outbreak of disease.
5   The causal agent should be re-isolated from the test host into pure culture and should be shown to be identical with the micro-organism initially isolated.

Even today these rules are still relevant, although we now appreciate that they cannot be rigidly applied in their original form to all types of pathogens. The most important exceptions in plant pathology are those pathogens which cannot be grown in artificial culture, viz. the viruses and some biotrophic fungi. The problem of isolating viruses from their host plants is generally overcome by using indicator plants. These are alternative hosts which develop symptoms which are specific for a particular virus. Healthy specimens of the original host may then be re-inoculated. In addition, electron microscopy of plant sap or of purified crystalline samples of the virus, coupled with serological techniques, may be employed to investigate the type(s) of virus present at each step of the infection procedure. The application of Koch's rules to non-culturable fungal pathogens presents less serious problems because they produce spores. These can be removed from the host and used in re-inoculation experiments. In many instances, spore morphology is also a valuable aid to the identification of the inoculated and re-isolated pathogens.

Further difficulties in satisfying these postulates may be experienced in cases where symptoms result from mixed infections or when dealing with previously undescribed disease agents. Not long ago, few pathologists would have predicted the existence of pathogens such as the viroids, which scarcely conform to our preconceptions of a successful parasite (see Chapter 4).

HOST RESISTANCE AND PATHOGEN VIRULENCE

Some crop plants are particularly prone to disease. For example tomatoes, potatoes, strawberries and tobacco are attacked by literally hundreds of different pathogens. In contrast other plants, such as cabbage, barley, sugar cane and pine trees, are infected by relatively few micro-organisms. These variations in disease occurrence are not, of course, entirely due to the distribution and frequency of pathogens. All crops are exposed to a range of infective propagules which are present both in soil and in the air. As a result, potato blight sporangia will land on lettuces, and cereal rust urediospores on oak leaves. Similarly, wheat roots grow into contact with *Plasmodiophora* resting spores. But none of these plants ever becomes affected by these particular pathogens.

These variations in the response of different crop species to particular pathogens are paralleled by differences in the responses of individuals within a host population. Even when a highly inbred crop cultivar is attacked by a specific pathogen, individual plants will vary in the severity of the symptoms which they develop.

All these variations reflect differences in the genetic constitution of both the host and the pathogen. Host response to pathogen invasion and the ability of the pathogen to cause disease have been shown to be determined by specific genes. This discovery has important implications both in the analysis of disease and in its control.

Resistance and susceptibility

When a micro-organism makes contact with a plant it may be able to penetrate the potential host or it may be completely excluded (Fig. 3.1). Following penetration, development of the pathogen may be quickly circumscribed by a host response or, alternatively, growth may continue within the host tissues.

Describing the interaction between a microbial pathogen and a plant host presents problems as the outcome needs to be defined in terms of both partners. At one extreme is the situation where a micro-organism is incapable of causing disease in the host under any conditions, and so is described as a non-pathogen of that host. Conversely, plants able to completely prevent penetration by a microbial agent are non-hosts, and are considered to be immune to that agent. The majority of interactions between microbes and green plants are likely to be of this type. It may, however, be difficult to establish whether a plant is immune to a particular pathogen, as the absence of visible symptoms does not automatically imply a failure to penetrate. Hence the use of the term immunity should be limited to cases where precise descriptions of the microbe–plant interactions are available.

In some instances, as will be described in more detail in Chapter 7, pathogens penetrate their hosts only to be immediately prevented from

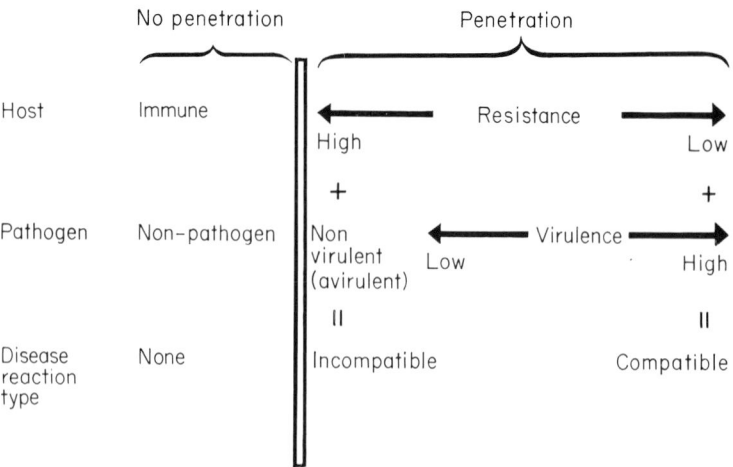

Figure 3.1 Relationship between host, pathogen and disease reaction. Note that the term immune, while being theoretically acceptable, raises many difficulties in practice—even in cases where there appears to be no disease reaction, penetration might have occurred. Similarly, non-pathogens have been shown to penetrate plants in which they are unable to establish a parasitic relationship.

further colonization by the death of the first living cells they enter. Such restricted development indicates that the host is RESISTANT to the pathogen. Resistance, unlike immunity, is not an all-or-nothing property of the host. In practice, there may be a whole range of responses. These vary from high resistance, where no visible symptoms are manifest, to low resistance, where the host completely succumbs to disease. Between these two extremes, resistance is described by a number of adjectives which though imprecise are of practical use in distinguishing between host reactions.

Alternatively, differing degrees of pathogen development may be described in terms of host susceptibility. For each degree of resistance there is a corresponding level of susceptibility. For instance, high resistance is equivalent to low susceptibility. Complete susceptibility is of considerable biological interest, as it appears to constitute the exception to the general rule that plants exhibit a degree of resistance. However, in this book we will normally consider these complementary descriptions of host responses only in terms of resistance. This approach has significant practical advantages in that it emphasizes the character which is selected for by plant breeders.

The terms resistance and susceptibility describe conditions of the host. However, just as the host may vary in its ability to resist infection so pathogens differ in their ability to invade and cause disease. Those micro-organisms which cannot enter a host are regarded as non-pathogenic with respect to that host. Others which are able to penetrate may be NON-VIRULENT (also termed avirulent), in that they have insignificant effects on the host; where the effects are more drastic they are described as possessing various degrees of virulence.

Genetic control of resistance and virulence

In common with all other biological characteristics, host resistance and pathogen virulence are genetically determined. However, these two properties can only be assessed in the presence of the other partner. In the majority of cases resistance or virulence is not obviously correlated with other phenotypic characters. Features of the pathogen, such as a rapid extension growth rate or the production of cell wall-degrading enzymes, may or may not be related to virulence. The interpretation of host resistance and pathogen virulence is therefore based on disease reaction types. The outcome of interactions between a highly resistant host and a non-virulent pathogen or between a host with low resistance and a highly virulent pathogen must be adequately described. An interaction where disease develops is described as a COMPATIBLE disease reaction whereas the opposite result constitutes an INCOMPATIBLE reaction (Fig. 3.1). An alternative way of describing these differences in disease expression is as high infection types and low infection types respectively.

Host resistance is controlled by one or a few genes whose individual effects may be easily detected, or by a multiplicity of genes, each of which contributes only a small fraction of the property as a whole. Resistance based on a limited number of genes is termed OLIGOGENIC (or monogenic if literally only one gene is involved) whereas resistance based on many genes is POLYGENIC. The closely related terms major gene resistance and minor gene resistance have sometimes been regarded as synonymous with oligogenic and polygenic but to avoid confusion their use is not recommended here (see p. 199).

Although pathogen virulence, host resistance and disease reaction types are genetically determined, the environment may modify the expression of any of these characters. For example, the *Sr6* gene conferring resistance in wheat to black stem rust is effective at 20°C but is rendered inoperative at 25°C.

In a few instances, resistance has been shown to be controlled by factors inherited through the host's cytoplasm. The best-known example of such cytoplasmically-determined resistance involves the reaction of maize to *Helminthosporium maydis*. The production of hybrid maize has in the past involved the laborious task of detasselling by hand to avoid self-pollination occurring. The discovery of a cytoplasmically inherited factor for male sterility, which meant that cross-pollination was essential, removed the need for this operation. Because of this, cultivars possessing male sterility factors came to predominate throughout the U.S.A. Unfortunately these sterility factors were also correlated with low resistance to *H. maydis*. As a result, the occurrence in 1970 of favourable conditions for the development of the disease resulted in a disastrous epidemic (see Fig. 6.8). In any breeding programme, the possibility that the cytoplasm may be important in disease resistance must therefore be considered.

Gene-for-gene theory

From an evolutionary viewpoint it is predictable that genetic systems determining virulence in the pathogen will be paralleled by genes conferring resistance in the host. This is because any mutation to virulence in a pathogen population will be countered by the selection of hosts able to resist this more aggressive pathogen. Thus, in an ideal world we might envisage a perpetual stalemate, with host and pathogen populations being closely matched in resistance and virulence. Hence over a period of several years disease would be neither completely absent nor would it become rampant.

Support for these ideas has been obtained by field observations and experimental studies on a limited number of host–pathogen combinations. Notable amongst these studies is the work of Flor on flax rust. He has shown that for each host gene conferring resistance there is a complementary gene in the pathogen determining virulence. This finding has become widely known as the GENE-FOR-GENE THEORY of host–pathogen interactions. More recently it has been pointed out that this system is more likely to operate in cases where resistance is determined by one or a few genes. On the basis of Flor's gene-for-gene theory, the possible interactions between a pair of alleles governing resistance in a plant and the corresponding pair determining virulence in the pathogen can be shown in the form of Fig. 3.2. In this quadratic check, a resistant reaction only occurs where an allele for resistance in the host plant interacts with an allele for avirulence in the pathogen.

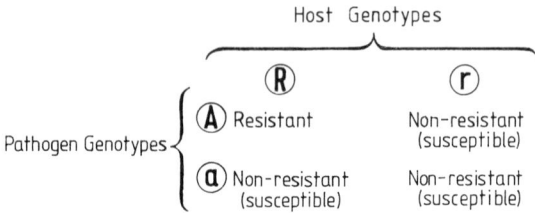

Figure 3.2 Possible interactions between alleles of a host resistance gene and a pathogen gene for virulence. Resistance R and avirulence A are normally dominant.

The gene-for-gene theory has important practical implications. The planting of crop cultivars containing a limited number of specific resistance genes will select out virulent strains of the pathogen. These strains are called RACES. The races present in any one season or in a particular locality may be identified by their reactions on a selection of cultivars carrying different combinations of genes conferring resistance.

Such differential reactions can be seen in a number of host–pathogen combinations. For example the resistance of tomatoes to leaf mould, caused by *Fulvia (Cladosporium) fulva*, is determined by four independent genes designated Cf 1, Cf 2, Cf 3 and Cf 4. The dominant allele of each gene confers resistance to some races of the pathogen but is ineffective against

Table 3.3 Reaction between some tomato cultivars and races of *Fulvia fulva* (data from Kaars Sijpesteijn & van Dijkman, 1973).

Tomato cultivar	Dominant resistance genes	Race of *Fulvia fulva*					
		o	1	2	4	1.2	1.2.4
Moneymaker	None	N	N	N	N	N	N
LMR	Cf1	R	N	R	R	N	N
Vetomold	Cf2	R	R	N	R	N	N
V473	Cf1, Cf2	R	R	R	R	N	N
Purdue 135	Cf4	R	R	R	N	R	N
Vagabond	Cf2, Cf4	R	R	R	R	R	N

R = Resistant, N = Non-resistant (Susceptible)

others. Table 3.3 lists some tomato cultivars containing different resistance genes or combinations of genes and shows the disease reaction which occurs between these cultivars and various races of the pathogen. Notation of the races in this instance indicates which resistance genes they can overcome.

In recent years plant breeders have introduced whole series of improved cultivars of many of our most important crops. Each new cultivar has tended to supercede its predecessor over most of the region where the crop is grown. The sequential introduction of these new cultivars has been accompanied by corresponding changes in pathogen populations whereby new races have successively come to predominate. The practical implications of this will be discussed in Chapter 10.

FURTHER READING

General texts

COOKE R.C. (1977) *The Biology of Symbiotic Fungi.* John Wiley & Sons, London.
An ambitious attempt to unravel the complexities of modes of nutrition of fungi, with a substantial number of references to parasitism.
DAY P.R. (1974) *Genetics of Host–Parasite Interaction.* W.H. Freeman, San Francisco.
A wide-ranging account which emphasises the genetic relationships between crops and their pathogens.
REID R. (1974) *Microbes and Men.* BBC Publications, London.
An entertaining history of the development of the germ theory of disease, with the emphasis on animal pathogens.

Reviews

COOKE R.C. & WHIPPS J.M. (1980) Evolution of modes of nutrition in fungi parasitic on terrestrial plants. *Biological Reviews* **55**, 341–362.
DAY P.R. (1981) Genetics of pathogenic fungi. *Symposium of the Society of General Microbiology* **31**, 361–378.
FLOR H.H. (1971) Current status of the gene for gene hypothesis. *Annual Review of Phytopathology* **9**, 275–296.
LEWIS D.H. (1973). Concepts in fungal nutrition and the origin of biotrophy. *Biological Reviews* **48**, 261–278.

4 Pathogen structure and function

"Scarcely any part of the organised world is free from the attack of parasites, a provision which is clearly one amongst many ordered by the Creator to maintain that balance amongst living beings . . ."

REV. M.J. BERKELEY (1803–1889)

By virtue of their life-style parasites are faced with a number of problems which, though not unique, are nevertheless more acute than those confronting free-living organisms. We have already seen that the evolution of biotrophy entails an increasing specialization to a narrow spectrum of hosts. An inevitable consequence of this increasing host specificity is that efficient colonization, reproduction, dispersal and survival assume even greater importance. It is hardly surprising, therefore, that parasitic micro-organisms have evolved a remarkable range of mechanisms which ensure their dispersal and survival.

A fundamental feature of all parasites is that the habitat itself is a living and genetically variable population of organisms. The genetic flexibility of micro-organisms, combined with their capacity for prolific reproduction, ensures, however, that by rapid evolution they maintain their status as successful parasites. Due to these features the microbial parasites are able to exploit many of the niches afforded by the breathtaking diversity of green plants in natural communities.

MORPHOLOGY AND GROWTH OF FUNGI, BACTERIA AND VIRUSES

The four groups of micro-organisms with which we are mainly concerned, the fungi, bacteria. mycoplasmas and viruses, have certain features in common as plant pathogens. For instance, they are all capable of rapid reproduction which results in the formation of numerous infective particles, known as propagules. Each group has, however, a distinctive and characteristic vegetative morphology (Fig. 4.1). These differences in vegetative form have important implications as regards their behaviour as plant pathogens.

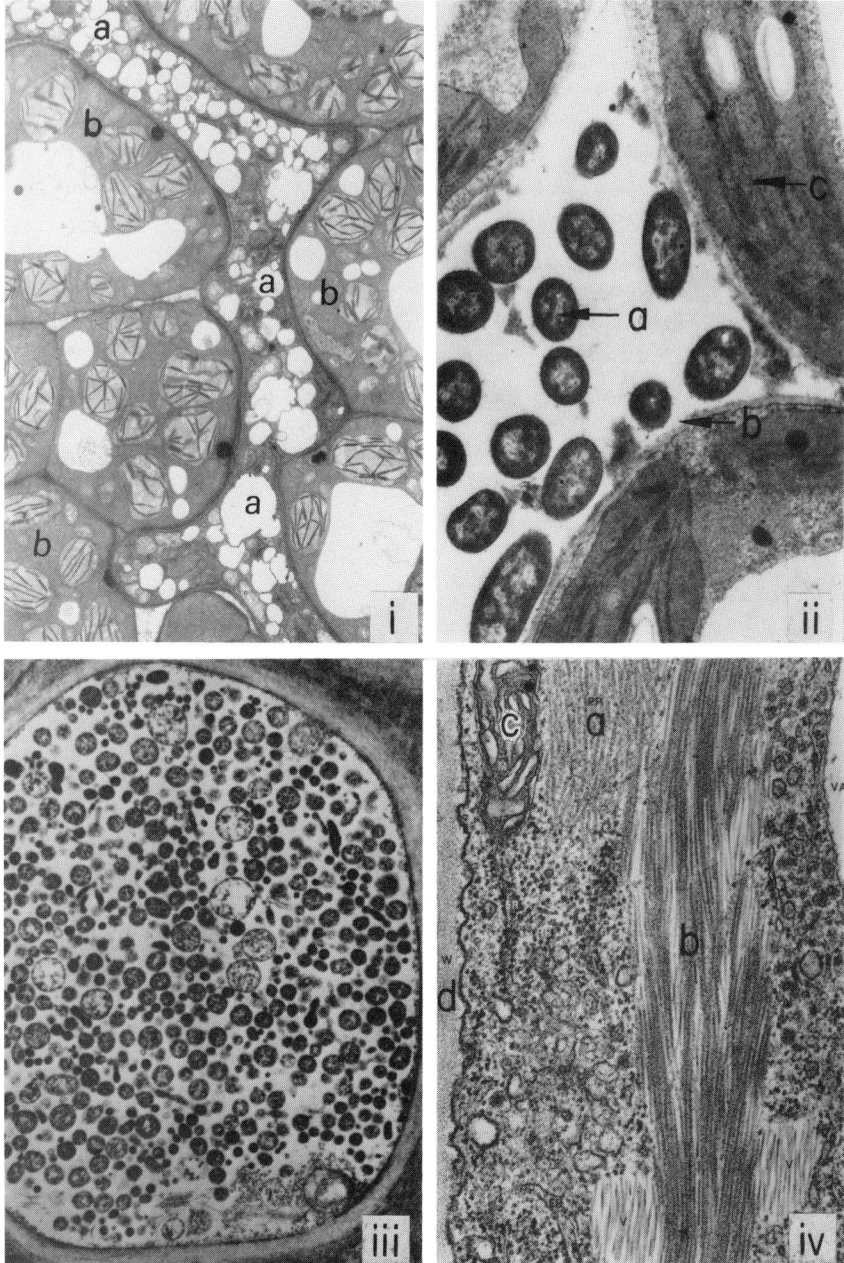

Figure 4.1 (i) Intercellular hypha of *Peronospora viciae* (*P. pisi*) in submeristematic shoot tissue of pea (× 3000) showing fungal hyphae (a) growing between host cells (b) which contain developing chloroplasts. The dark deposits in host cells adjacent to hyphae mark sites at which intracellular haustoria will develop. (ii) *Pseudomonas phaseolicola* cells in an intercellular space in a French bean leaf (× 12 700) showing bacterial cells (a), host cell walls (b), and host cytoplasm containing chloroplasts (c). (iii) Mycoplasma-like bodies in sieve tube of *Nicotiana rustica* (× 11 050) showing the variable morphology of these organisms. (iv) Tobacco mosaic virus in phloem parenchyma cell of tobacco (× 67 500) showing striate crystalline aggregates of the virus in various orientations (a, b), a host cell mitochondrion (c), and the host cell wall (d). Photographs from: (i) Hickey & Coffey, 1977; (ii) Sigee & Epton; (iii) Hirumi & Maramorosch, 1973; (iv) Esau, 1968.

Fungi

Most plant-pathogenic fungi form HYPHAE (singular = hypha), that is tubular thalli, which extend by apical growth and an ordered system of branching. The network of hyphae which results from such growth is called a MYCELIUM, and the interconnected mycelium derived from one propagule or resulting from the fusion of hyphae from two or more propagules is termed a COLONY.

As a hypha grows through the substrate it secretes extracellular enzymes which digest complex molecules. The products of this process are then absorbed by the hypha. Not all filamentous fungi have the same enzymatic capabilities. For example, many heart-rot pathogens secrete cellulase and ligninases which enable them to utilize the complex constituents of wood. In contrast, many of the pathogens which attack herbaceous tissues are noted for their production of pectolytic enzymes.

The relationship between growing hyphal tips and the older, first-formed parts of the colony varies at different stages in the life cycle of a fungus. Three different patterns of behaviour may be identified. In some fungi, as hyphae extend at their apices the older portions of the colony become moribund and may autolyse, or be destroyed by bacteria or grazing animals. Amongst pathogenic fungi, this type of growth is found in *Pythium* and *Rhizopus*. Sporulation in these fungi occurs at or near the advancing margin of the colony. Following disintegration of the first-formed hyphae the older parts of the lesion are quickly invaded by secondary organisms.

The hyphae of other fungi are longer-lived. They can act as transport systems from the older parts of the colony to the hyphal tips. Such transport systems are probably not important while the pathogen is still colonizing the original host, but they are often essential when fungi attempt to grow from one host to another. Unless the fungus is then able to obtain nutrients in competition with saprophytic micro-organisms, it must fuel both its growth across inhospitable terrain and the subsequent infection processes needed to establish itself on a new host, by transporting nutrients from its established food base. Hyphae growing on the surface or away from their host face problems due to adverse environmental factors, particularly desiccation and the destructive activities of the associated microfauna. Hyphae may therefore exhibit adaptations which improve their efficiency and success in this role. The RUNNER HYPHAE of *Gaeumannomyces graminis*, which facilitate rapid and extensive growth along the surface of roots, have thicker, darker-coloured walls than those hyphae involved in penetration and colonization of individual parts of the host's tissues. Other fungi produce aggregate structures consisting of a number of hyphae grouped together. At their simplest, these form MYCELIAL STRANDS within which there is relatively little differentiation. In more massive and elaborate structures known as RHIZOMORPHS the outermost hyphae, which have thickened and pigmented walls, form a resistant rind while the internal hyphae are differentiated into a highly efficient transporting system. Rhizomorphs can grow five to six times faster than normal vegetative hyphae. They are formed by many tree pathogens, such as *Armillaria mellea* and *Fomes lignosus*.

The third type of colonial behaviour is exhibited by the rust fungi and several other biotrophic pathogens. In these the whole colony remains functional for a relatively long period and transport of nutrients takes place from the advancing colony margin to the centre, where there is usually some continuing activity such as sporulation. Rust fungi develop these integrated colonies within photosynthetic tissues and the continuing activity of their colonies depends on the host tissues remaining viable.

Individual hyphae are frequently modified in form to accomplish particular functions, and this is especially common amongst pathogenic species. The problems encountered in the infection and colonization of a host have in many cases been surmounted by the evolution of specialized hyphal structures. Appressoria, infection hyphae and haustoria (Fig. 4.2) are all examples of such hyphal adaptations (see Chapter 5).

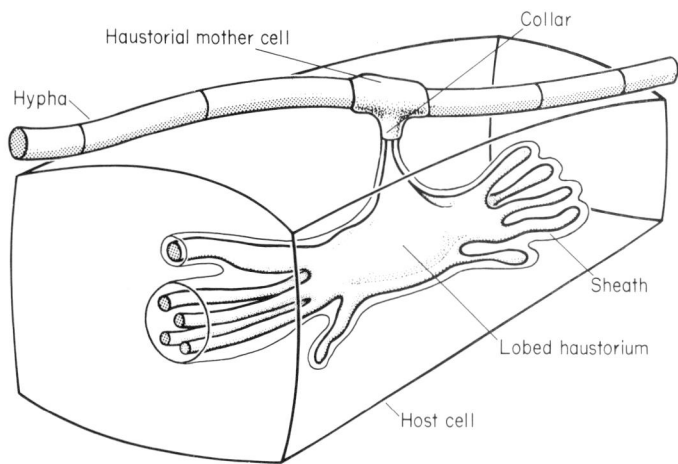

Figure 4.2 *Erysiphe* haustorium in an epidermal cell (adapted from Bracker, 1968).

Bacteria

In most species of plant-pathogenic bacteria, cell division is by binary fission and the subsequent activities of the separated cells are not coordinated in any way. The major exceptions to this generalization are the bacterial pathogens classified in the Actinomycetales. *Streptomyces* and *Actinomyces*, for example, form a rudimentary branching mycelium composed of relatively narrow, septate filaments. Sometimes individual bacterial cells aggregate to form substantial colonies, as in crown gall or in the cankers resulting from fireblight infection. In other cases, however, cells spread throughout an entire organ or physiological system. Soft-rot bacteria in potatoes spread indiscriminately through tuber tissues, while vascular wilt bacteria in cucurbits are widely dispersed within the host's xylem. Growth of single-celled bacteria, like fungi, also involves the production of extracellular enzymes.

However, most plant-pathogenic bacteria are not able to degrade complex substances, such as cellulose and lignin. There is less integration in the development of a colony (which may be defined as the sum total of cells originating from one individual) than is possible in fungi. Actinomycete colonies are probably comparable with those of the damping-off fungi, but we still know little about the biology of these organisms. Neither the filamentous forms nor the more numerous single-celled bacteria are able to produce modified cells to facilitate penetration into or spread within host plants.

Mycoplasmas

In recent years it has become evident that a number of diseases once thought to be of viral aetiology are in fact caused by a group of prokaryotic organisms known as mycoplasmas. In particular, several yellows diseases, characterized by extensive chlorosis and a gradual decline in the host, are associated with the presence of large numbers of these organisms in the phloem. Despite their superficial similarity in electronmicrographs of infected tissue, it is now clear that this group includes two different types of agent, the true mycoplasmas and the spiroplasmas. Both types may be regarded as bacteria which have lost the ability to form a rigid cell wall; they are highly pleomorphic, and it seems probable that under natural conditions they cannot survive apart from their hosts or vectors. Mycoplasmas are similar to viruses in their inability to form penetration structures or to multiply outside host cells, and is being transmitted by grafting and by dodder or insect vectors. They are susceptible to tetracyclines and treatment of the host with these antibiotics leads to remission of symptoms.

The spiroplasmas have now been successfully cultured on artificial media in which they typically assume a motile, helical form (Fig. 4.3). To date, no true mycoplasma has been cultured away from its host or vector.

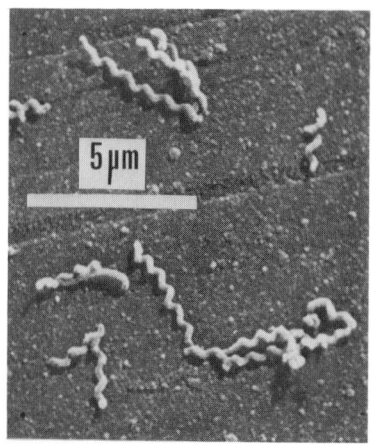

Figure 4.3 Scanning electronmicrograph of *Spiroplasma* cells from a pure culture (photograph by courtesy of P.G. Markham, R. Townsend & J. Burgess, John Innes Institute).

A number of very destructive diseases are now known to be caused by mycoplasmas. Coconut lethal yellowing (which has virtually destroyed the industry in the Caribbean), corn stunt and citrus stubborn have all been attributed to mycoplasma-like organisms. There is little doubt that, as more diseases presently assumed to be caused by viruses are subjected to rigorous analysis, mycoplasmas will assume greater importance as plant pathogens.

Viruses

The ultimate simplicity in vegetative morphology is found in the viruses. These are non-cellular, consisting of a nucleic acid core surrounded by a protein coat or capsid and occur either as individual particles or as crystalline aggregates within cells. In comparison with fungi and bacteria, the viruses appear extremely ill-equipped to act as pathogens, due to their inability to grow outside living cells. However, their extreme specialization and efficient replication once established inside a host, together with their elegant and efficient dispersal methods, ensure that they are successful and potentially devastating plant pathogens.

Viral parasitism is unique, in that the parasite itself is incorporated into the metabolism of the host cell. After gaining entry into a living cell, the nucleic acid component of the virus is released from its protein coat. The viral genome is then translated and replicated, and numerous new virus particles are assembled from the newly synthesized nucleic acid and protein. In contrast to fungi and bacteria, viruses do not attack the structural integrity of their host tissues but instead exploit the synthetic machinery of the host cell and divert energy to their own ends.

Five classes of plant virus have been described, containing a DNA or RNA genome in either double-stranded or single-stranded form; where the nucleic acid is single-stranded, the polarity of the strand may be the same as messenger RNA or complementary to it. The precise sequence of events during replication within the host cell is determined by the type of nucleic acid present (see *Introduction to Modern Virology*, Volume 2 in the Basic Microbiology series). The majority of plant viruses contain a single strand of RNA which, once freed from its coat protein, can act directly as messenger RNA in the synthesis of further virus particles. This messenger must code for at least two components, an RNA replicase enzyme and new virus-coat protein. Evidence from bacterial viruses indicates that the replicase enzyme may in fact contain subunits of host origin, as well as those coded for by the virus. A double-stranded form of RNA has been detected in virus-infected plant cells; the existence of this 'replicative form' suggests that the viral RNA acts as a template for its complementary strand, which then in turn acts as a template for new strands of viral RNA.

In other plant viruses, the viral nucleic acid must first be transcribed to yield messenger RNA, from either an RNA or DNA template. The polymerase enzyme necessary to achieve this transcription may already be present in the intact virus particle.

Viroids

Viroids differ from viruses in the size of their RNA genomes and in their lack of an associated protein coat. These free RNA molecules have a molecular weight of *c.* 120 000, which is at least ten times smaller than a typical RNA-virus genome. This amount of genetic information appears to be minimal, and insufficient to code for even a single enzyme. This raises the interesting question as to how these agents modify host cells to cause disease.

The first disease definitely attributed to a viroid was potato spindle tuber and the complete nucleotide sequence of this RNA is now known (see Gross *et al.*, 1978). At least four other diseases are known to be caused by viroids.

Conclusions

What is the importance of these groups of organisms in pathology? Most notorious diseases of man and other animals are caused by bacteria and viruses. By contrast, plants are more commonly affected by fungi and viruses. This difference in the significance of particular groups of micro-organisms can be explained on the basis of several basic differences between plants and animals (Table 4.1). Bacteria generally favour warm,

Table 4.1 Higher plants and animals compared as hosts.

Plants	Animals
Anatomical features	
Rigid cell wall	No cell wall
No circulatory system	Circulatory system
Internal environment	
Acid pH	Alkaline pH
High C/N ratio	Low C/N ratio
No temperature regulation	Temperature regulation

alkaline conditions with high nitrogen levels. Being unicellular, effective spread within the host is enhanced by a circulatory system. Filamentous fungi are more effective parasites of higher plants as their requirements are generally in direct contrast to those of bacteria. While these generalizations appear to hold good today, the extent to which such preferences are due to progressive adaptation to animal or plant hosts is not known.

PATHOGEN REPRODUCTION AND VARIATION

Micro-organisms are capable of extremely rapid reproduction and they form astronomical numbers of propagules. In single-celled organisms growth automatically leads to early cell division and cell separation. In the majority of the fungi there is an initial period of vegetative growth prior to the formation of reproductive propagules termed spores. Even so, sporulation may commence shortly after infection and enormous numbers of spores are rapidly formed.

In conventional biological terms, reproduction can be classified as either sexual or asexual. Sexual reproduction involves meiosis and the subsequent fusion of compatible nuclei contained within gametes or other sexual structures. Asexual reproduction is a simple replication of the organism based on mitotic divisions of nuclei. This process does not offer the same possibilities of genetic recombination, and hence of variation in populations, as sexual systems.

Amongst micro-organisms, however, such clear-cut distinctions in reproductive processes are not always readily discerned. The mode of replication of virus particles within host cells is not strictly comparable with division in the cellular micro-organisms. However, in terms of pathogen multiplication and spread the end result is similar. Variation is demonstrable in virus populations and this must in some way be linked with reproduction in the host cell.

Bacteria

The bacteria are the best-known examples of single-celled organisms which maintain their form by regular binary fission and separation of daughter cells. Bacteria also reproduce sexually, but less frequently than the fungi. Owing to their normal haploid state and the absence of a clearly defined nucleus, this process is more irregular than is found elsewhere in the plant and animal kingdoms. DNA passes from one cell, the donor, to another, the recipient, by transduction, transformation or conjugation. Transduction, which is mediated by bacteriophages, is possibly the most common method in nature.

Fungi

The fungi exhibit a very wide range of reproductive mechanisms. Asexual reproduction seems to be of prime importance in increasing the number of individuals. Epidemic spread of pathogens usually depends on the production of countless asexual spores. The Mastigomycotina and the Zygomycotina form asexual spores in SPORANGIA and these can themselves function as propagules or alternatively release a number of motile zoospores or non-motile aplanospores. The asexual spores of the Ascomycotina and Basidiomycotina are termed CONIDIA. However, some of these fungi, especially those Basidiomycotina which form large sexual fruit bodies, reproduce asexually only very rarely, if at all.

Sexual reproduction is a regular occurrence in the life histories of many fungal pathogens, such as *Armillaria mellea, Claviceps purpurea* and *Peronospora parasitica*. In many instances it fulfils a dual role of increasing variation in the population and ensuring survival through unfavourable periods. In some species, however, it is apparently an exceptional or very rare event. In fact, one group of fungi, the Fungi Imperfecti (or

Deuteromycotina), is defined on the basis of the absence or infrequency of sexual reproduction. *Penicillium* on citrus fruits, *Botrytis* on strawberries and *Fulvia* on tomatoes are all examples of pathogens which seem to have relegated sexual reproduction to a minor role in their biology. Even when sexual reproduction is a regular feature of a fungal life cycle, it usually only occurs under a more limited range of host and environmental conditions than permit asexual reproduction.

The nature of sexual reproduction varies considerably among the major groups of fungi. Four main types of sexual spore can be identified, each being characteristic of one of the major groups of fungi. Thus OOSPORES, ZYGOSPORES, ASCOSPORES and BASIDIOSPORES are formed by the Mastigomycotina, the Zygomycotina, the Ascomycotina and the Basidiomycotina respectively. Sexual spores sometimes germinate quickly, as in the case of *Puccinia* basidiospores on barberry or *Claviceps* ascospores on grass stigmata. In these fungi, the survival function has usually been accomplished prior to spore formation, by the perennation of dormant survival structures. In contrast, the oospores formed by the lower fungi can remain viable for extended periods even when exposed to environmental stresses.

Some economically important pathogens, notably the rusts, have extremely complex life cycles in which as many as five different types of spore participate in a regular sequence. A complete rust life cycle involves urediospores, teliospores, basidiospores, pycniospores and aeciospores. Epidemic spread is essentially due to urediospores, which are asexual conidia, whereas variation and survival are ensured by the other four types of spore.

Variation in populations

Variation in pathogen populations is maintained by several methods (Table 4.2). The relative importance of these different methods varies for the several types of microbial pathogens. Mutation is probably of equal significance in all groups. The sexual cycle is clearly important for many fungi and for some of the bacteria. Heterokaryosis (the occurrence of two or more genetically different nuclei in a common cytoplasm) and the parasexual cycle are peculiar to the fungi.

The parasexual cycle permits a degree of genetic recombination without the normal steps involved in sexual reproduction taking place (Fig. 4.4). It

Table 4.2 Mechanisms maintaining variation in pathogen populations. The more crosses, the more commonly the mechanism is used.

	Fungi	Bacteria	Virus
Sexual reproduction	+ + +	+	−
Heterokaryosis	+ + +	−	−
Parasexual cycle	+ + +	−	−
Mutation	+	+	+ +
Cytoplasmic factors	+ +	+ + +	−

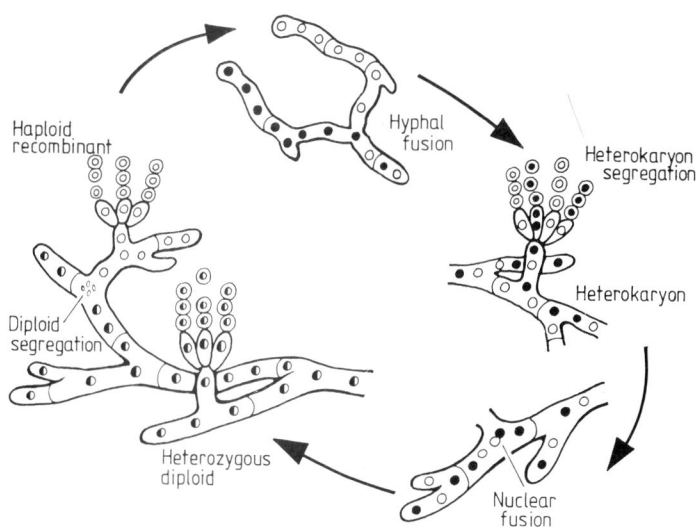

Figure 4.4 The parasexual cycle (after Sermonti, 1977).

must be emphasized that for any species this phenomenon only occurs during the formation of a tiny percentage of its asexual spores, but as literally millions of asexual spores are produced the parasexual cycle assumes considerable significance. Cytoplasmic factors are only able to operate in the bacteria and fungi.

There is an increasing body of evidence which suggests that extra-chromosomal genetic elements, known as PLASMIDS, play an important role in determining the virulence of pathogenic bacteria. For instance, with some animal pathogens, the abilities to adhere to host cells and to elaborate toxins may both be plasmid-coded traits. Less information is currently available for plant-pathogenic bacteria, with the striking exception of *Agrobacterium tumefaciens*, the causal agent of crown gall disease (see p. 142).

These mechanisms ensure that in natural environments pathogen populations encompass a range of variation which enables them to contend with changes in their hosts or in the environment. Indeed, the apparently endless capacity for variation amongst pathogens remains a major stumbling block in man's search for disease-resistant crops.

DISPERSAL OF PATHOGENS

Colonization of a particular habitat is inexorably followed sooner or later by spread, as space and nutrients become limiting. The problem of dispersal is by no means peculiar to pathogens. It is, on the contrary, a fundamental feature of the life cycle of all living organisms. However, because of their adaptation to a narrow ecological niche, namely a living host, an especially efficient means of dispersal is a basic requirement for pathogens.

Although dispersal is usually thought of in terms of spatial spread, it should be borne in mind that the time scale over which this spread takes place is an important consideration. While dispersal may take only a few hours or even minutes, in other cases a slow spread may occur over a number of years.

Many pathogens spread through crops in a spectacular manner. Some cover tremendous distances at remarkable speeds. In general, the most dramatic examples of spread involve pathogens with air-borne propagules (Fig. 4.5). Pathogens which infect subterranean organs often exhibit a

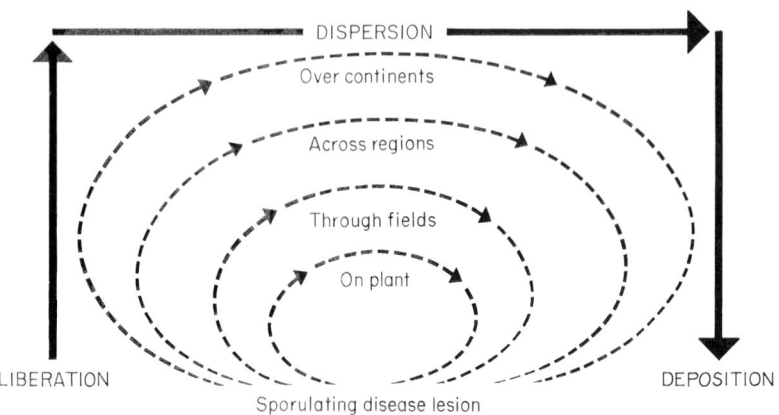

Figure 4.5 The processes involved in pathogen dispersal and the scale on which they operate.

restricted pattern of dispersal through the soil. These generalizations apply particularly to the pathogens which have developed their own independent processes for dispersal. Organisms which rely on vectors are at the mercy of these transport systems, in respect of the distances and speeds achieved. Man must be included here as an often-unwitting vector who can radically alter normal patterns of pathogen distribution. He is especially important when he aids and abets a pathogen which is normally dependent upon its host's own dispersal processes. Seed-borne pathogens provide obvious examples here but there are also well-established instances of pathogens being transported in all the types of vegetative organs used in plant propagation.

There are almost as many dispersal mechanisms as there are pathogens. Some of these mechanisms are both elegant and highly efficient in that they are closely adapted to the biology of the host. The synchronization of spore release in certain pathogens, e.g. *Venturia* and *Claviceps*, with bud-break or flowering increases the chances of propagules finding vulnerable host tissues. Other pathogens merely saturate the environment with propagules in an apparently haphazard and wasteful manner. The fruit bodies of bracket fungi causing heart rots release literally billions of spores over several months.

We do not propose merely to list examples of dispersal mechanisms but rather we shall consider the four main routes of dispersal, namely via the aerial environment, through the soil, in vectors, and by man.

Aerial environment

Dispersal via the atmosphere involves three distinct phases, liberation of the propagules, dispersion and finally, deposition (Fig. 4.5). In the first phase the pathogen itself may participate actively but during the two latter processes propagules are transported passively.

Liberation has two aspects, the release of propagules from the parent colony and their take-off from the host surface. Take-off is of special interest as it involves the boundary layer phenomenon. This is a zone of still air which surrounds all surfaces including the soil, plant leaves, stems, petals, etc. and the crop canopy, inasmuch as this forms a definite layer. The thickness of the boundary layer varies according to a number of factors, particularly wind speed and turbulence and the size and shape of the surface.

Some pathogens, notably many fungi, have evolved sophisticated methods which enable their spores to pass through the boundary layer into the turbulent air beyond (Fig. 4.6). Many of these methods have been described in great detail by Ingold, who has commented on the elaborate ways in which they are related to the environment. Other pathogens, including

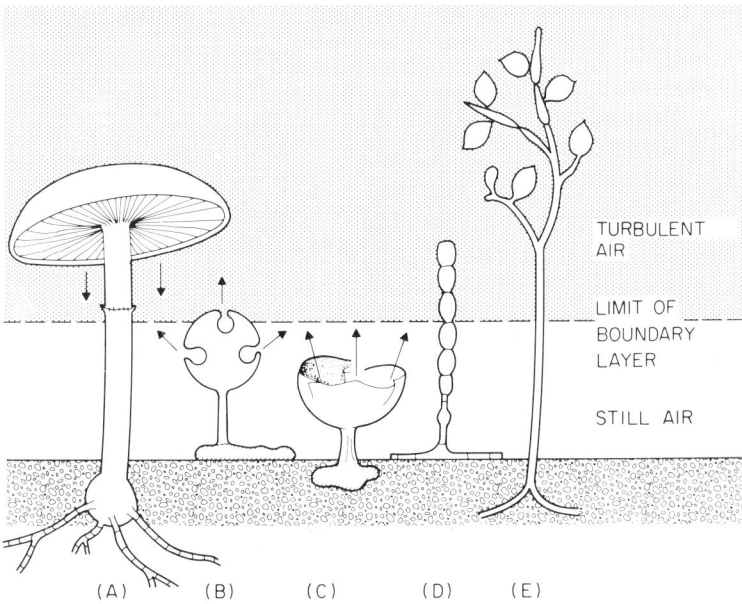

Figure 4.6 Devices employed by fungi to escape from the boundary layer. Gravity, (A) *Armillaria*; violent discharge, (B) *Claviceps* and (C) *Sclerotinia*; chain extension, (D) *Erysiphe*; long sporangiophores, (E) *Phytophthora*.

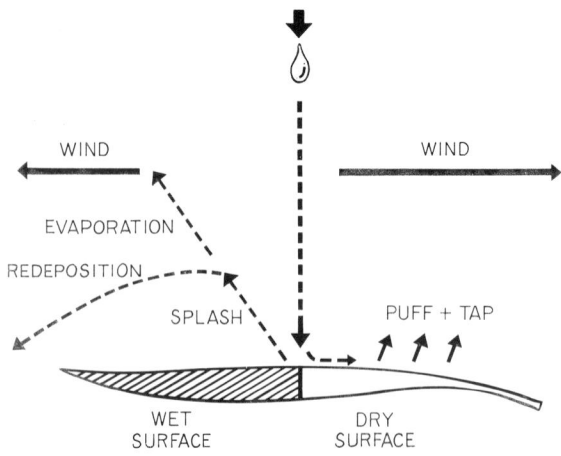

Figure 4.7 Spore dispersal by raindrops from wet and dry leaves.

many bacteria and some fungi, take advantage of external dispersal agencies. Foremost amongst these are rain drops which splash or puff and tap spores off from wet and dry surfaces respectively (Fig. 4.7). Gregory (1973) has emphasized the importance of rain drops as dispersal mechanisms. In regions with a rainfall of 100 cm per year (which is a normal amount for north-west Europe) each square metre of ground will be hit by about one thousand million rain drops. Each drop can break up into as many as 5000 splash droplets which may carry wettable spores through the boundary layer. These water droplets plus spores can bounce directly onto an adjacent plant or, if the water evaporates, the propagules can become truly air-borne. In addition to rain drops, wind, mist and convection currents can all act to liberate propagules under particular circumstances.

Liberation is followed by dispersal. This may be rapid and local, as when spores travel in splash drops, or conversely, it may involve transport in the upper atmosphere across continents over several weeks. Some really fascinating questions concerning this stage in the propagule's journey remain to be answered. Can spores cross the oceans? Do regular sequential disease outbreaks across a region signify the movement of a pathogen? What factors limit the survival of spores in the upper reaches of the earth's atmosphere?

Other unanswered questions concern the final stage of dispersal, i.e. deposition onto a plant surface. In calm conditions, diffusion brings spores into contact with the boundary layer. On entering this layer of still air they fall onto the surface under the influence of gravity. In windy conditions spores can be impacted onto objects which project into the air stream. This process is not, however, very efficient and it is only of any importance for large spores which become impacted on small, narrow surfaces at high wind speeds. The number of spores deposited in this way is increased if the air currents are turbulent.

Rain drops collect the air spora and deposit it on plant surfaces. Both large and small propagules are picked up by rain drops and they can be carried down from all levels of the atmosphere. Less is known about deposition due to electric charges or temperature gradients, but both may be important for some pathogens and/or crops.

Soil environment

Pathogens which only infect subterranean tissues are in a minority, but despite the obvious problems which they face regarding dispersal, many cause serious economic problems. *Plasmodiophora*, *Pythium* and *Fusarium* are examples of pathogens which thrive within the soil environment. Undoubtedly, time plays a more important part in dispersal for soil-borne pathogens than it does for their airborne counterparts. The pathogens causing the above diseases all form spores which can persist for long periods (see the section on Survival, pp. 51–8).

Patterns of spatial dispersal of soil-borne pathogens are generally restricted, at least in the short term. Some spread through crops only slowly, forming circular patches within which most if not all plants are infected. Other pathogens which primarily attack subterranean tissues are not so restricted. Some of these emerge briefly from below ground solely for the purpose of dispersal. *Gaeumannomyces* spreads by mycelial growth along roots in soil but it can also produce an annual crop of airborne ascospores from perithecia embedded in stubble. Ascospores were almost certainly responsible for the outbreaks of take-all on newly reclaimed polders in Holland. Other soil-borne pathogens are passively if irregularly dispersed as a result of wind or water erosion.

Whilst soil may not offer the same opportunities for dispersal as the aerial environment, it does in part compensate by providing a suitable medium for microbial growth. Amongst microbial pathogens only the fungi possess the capabilities to really exploit this advantage. Numerous studies have been made to determine the extent to which such growth occurs. Two interrelated problems are envisaged. The pathogen must be capable of obtaining nutrients to continue growth and it must also be able to withstand direct and indirect antagonism from the soil microflora and fauna. It has become clear that different fungi exhibit a wide range of capabilities for saprophytic growth in soil. Some, such as *Plasmodiophora*, scarcely grow at all away from the living host. At the other extreme, *Pythium* and *Rhizoctonia* are almost equally good saprophytes as they are parasites. This means that they are able to spread very widely in soil by hyphal growth.

Between these extremes there is one group of pathogens which, though not such efficient saprophytes as *Pythium*, are nevertheless able to spread effectively in soil. *Armillaria* and *Fomes* form rhizomorphs which grow along root surfaces and through soil for considerable distances. In this instance, nutrition is being supplied by the previously parasitized host rather than by the debris in the soil.

Considering the physical nature of soil it is not surprising that vectors are also exploited by a number of soil-borne pathogens. Reliance on vectors is not, however, confined to soil organisms and many of our comments on this subject are equally valid for any environment.

Vectors

A wide variety of animals and microbes feed on green plants. During their feeding activities many move from plant to plant, sometimes over long distances. Not surprisingly, pathogens exploit some of these organisms as agents of dispersal. Any organism which transmits or disperses a pathogen is termed a VECTOR. Some examples are shown in Fig. 4.8.

Three types of pathogen–vector relationship may be identified. In a few instances the relationship is highly specific. The pathogen continues to multiply within the vector and the behaviour of the vector is ideally suited to dispersal of the pathogen. These remarkably dovetailed patterns of behaviour have resulted in the creation of dispersal systems which are highly efficient. More commonly, multiplication of the pathogen does not take place within the vector which is merely contaminated internally or externally. However, a distinction may be made among these vectors according to

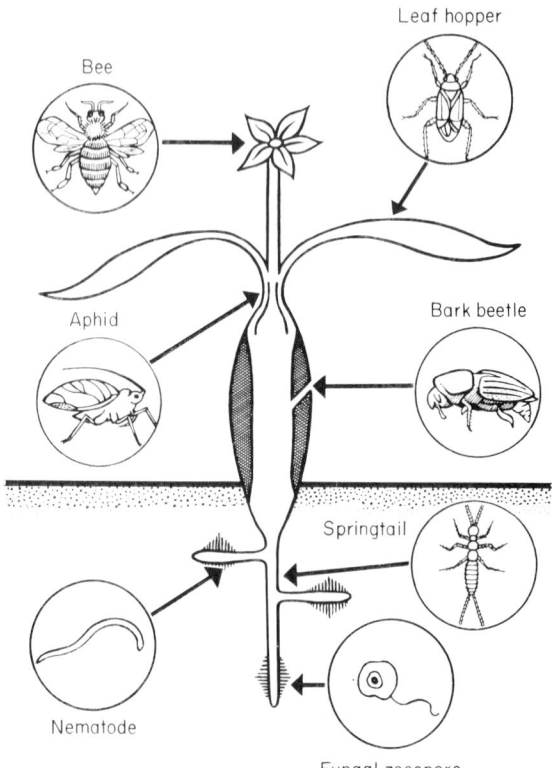

Figure 4.8 Vectors exploited by plant pathogens.

46

the extent to which their life style is matched with that of the pathogen. In the least integrated relationships the pathogen is spread sporadically by a variety of vectors, none of which is especially well suited to this task. Such chance contamination is often, however, important in the establishment of disease in new areas.

Vectors are frequently thought of as only being involved in the transmission of viruses. However, whilst it is true that vectors are of supreme importance in the life cycle of numerous viruses, it should also be emphasized that they are valuable or even essential for the dispersal of many bacteria and fungi. For example, *Erwinia amylovora* and *Ceratocystis ulmi* depend for their spread on pollinating insects and bark beetles respectively. Many fungi produce spores which can survive the digestive processes in animal guts. Ingestion and subsequent excretion may thus result in spores being dispersed and, incidentally, deposited within a nutritious faecal pellet. Vascular wilt fungi sporulate on the surface of dying roots, and soil animals have been seen grazing on the protruding hyphae and spores. Presumably the latter are then deposited randomly throughout the soil, which enhances their chance of encountering developing roots.

Virus vectors

Due to their morphological simplicity, many viruses have come to depend entirely upon vectors for their dispersal. Most of these vectors are also themselves pests or parasites, as contamination by the virus only takes place if the vector penetrates living cells. Thus aphids, leafhoppers, nematodes and even parasitic fungi are doubly important in that they carry one or more viruses, as well as themselves causing significant crop losses. The spectrum of relationships between viruses and their vectors, with particular reference to patterns of infectivity, is illustrated in Table 4.3.

Among all these vectors, most is known about the activities of the sapsucking insects which infest leaves and other photosynthetic tissues. Aphids and leafhoppers insert their stylets into the phloem and while extracting sap they also acquire virus particles. In some vectors this inoculum may be transferred immediately to another plant which the insect probes as a possible food source. The insect may then be free from virus until it again feeds on an affected plant. In other vectors contamination is followed by a more or less extended period during which the virus becomes established in the vector. The virus may or may not multiply in the vector, which is not infective until the end of this establishment phase. Subsequently, the vector is able to infect plants over an extended period, which in extreme cases covers the rest of its life. In some vectors infection may even be transmitted through eggs to the next generation.

The various relationships described in Table 4.3 appear to lead to a number of equally sophisticated and successful strategies which ensure the efficient spread and survival of the pathogens. These fascinating relationships have been the subject of a great deal of study and a number of alter-

Table 4.3 Strategies involved in virus–vector relationships.

	Persistence of virus in vector		
	Non-persistent (stylet-borne)*	Semi-persistent (stylet-borne)	Persistent (circulative, propagative/non-propagative)
Vectors	Aphids, chytrids, mites	Aphids, beetles, leafhoppers, mealy bugs, whiteflies	Aphids, beetles, bugs, fungi, leafhoppers, mites, nematodes, thrips, whiteflies
Location of virus in vector	Externally, on or near mouthparts	Near junction of stylet and tip	Internally, e.g. in haemolymph
Vector/virus specificity	Mostly low	Intermediate	Mostly high
Minimum time from acquisition of virus to inoculation of virus-free plant	Several seconds or minutes	30 min to several hours	12 hours to several days
Period during which vector remains infective	< 10 hours (usually < 4)	10–100 hours	> 100 hours
Multiplication of virus in vector	No	No	Yes, in some instances

* Refer to those members of the fauna which have appropriate mouthparts.

native schemes of classification have been proposed to provide a framework for further discussion. One such scheme emphasises the location of the virus in the vector, with some being described as stylet-borne and others as circulative. These categories approximate to non-persistent and persistent respectively, but as it is not known for certain where the virus particles are actually located in most vectors, the scheme outlined in Table 4.3 is preferred for use in this book.

Whereas most vectors operate in the aerial environment a few viruses are dispersed through the soil by nematodes and parasitic fungi. Fan leaf in grapevine and ringspot in raspberry are two examples of viruses spread by nematodes which themselves feed on living plant roots. Lettuce big vein and tobacco stunt viruses are transmitted by *Olpidium*, a parasitic, root-infecting chytrid. Recent developments in horticultural practice, in which plants are grown in a circulating liquid film of nutrients, have provided extremely favourable opportunities for the rapid and extensive dispersal of the chytrid zoospores which carry these viruses.

Two particularly interesting routes of virus dispersal involve the parasitic plant dodder and transmission in pollen. Dodder has been used experimentally to transmit viruses between different host species but it is doubtful if it is of any practical significance under field conditions. Pollen offers a potentially ideal route for virus spread, because it becomes widely dispersed and the virus need never be exposed to the external environment. Contaminated pollen may transmit virus through the stigma to either the seed parent or the seed or both. From an agricultural viewpoint it is perhaps fortunate that such an efficient transmission system is uncommon. Amongst cases which are known are a number of fruit crop viruses such as prunus necrotic ringspot and raspberry bushy dwarf which are both spread effectively as a result of cross-pollination from affected plants.

In those viruses which are seed-borne it appears that contamination of the seed from the pollen is as important as contamination from the mother plant, with both processes occurring with equal frequency in most cases of seed-transmitted viruses.

Man as a vector

Aside from natural vectors and the other dispersal mechanisms discussed so far it is necessary to consider the impact of man on this aspect of pathology. His activities fall under two main headings; he has exaggerated the significance of some naturally occurring dispersal mechanisms and he himself has become a new super-vector with remarkable potential.

Man has substantially increased the threat posed by seed-borne disease. Seeds naturally constitute a very important dispersal mechanism for pathogens; all seeds may harbour a wide variety of pathogens which are either established internally or are mere surface contaminants. For example, soybean seeds can carry a remarkable variety of pathogens as indicated in Fig. 4.9. Seeds of crop plants are no longer dispersed naturally, but are the

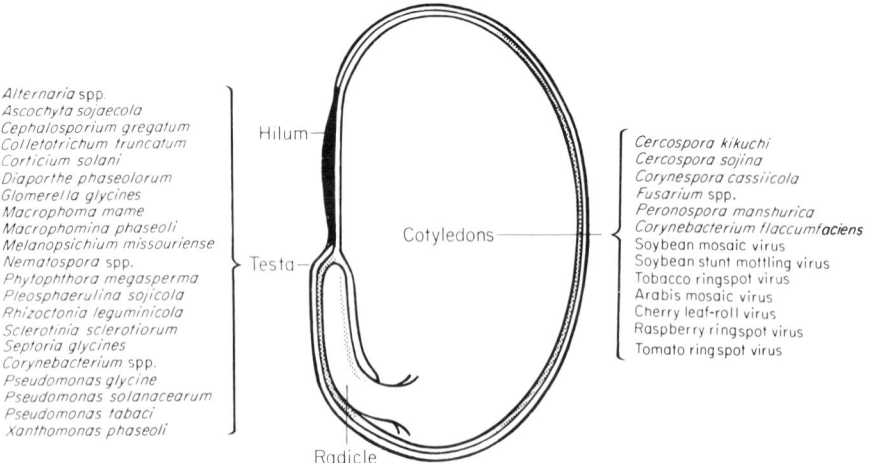

Figure 4.9 Pathogens known to be dispersed on or in soybean seed. Most of these pathogens are omitted from the appendix.

The labelled pathogen lists in the figure read:

Left list:
Alternaria spp.
Ascochyta sojaecola
Cephalosporium gregatum
Colletotrichum truncatum
Corticium solani
Diaporthe phaseolorum
Glomerella glycines
Macrophoma mame
Macrophomina phaseoli
Melanopsichium missouriense
Nematospora spp.
Phytophthora megasperma
Pleosphaerulina sojicola
Rhizoctonia leguminicola
Sclerotinia sclerotiorum
Septoria glycines
Corynebacterium spp.
Pseudomonas glycine
Pseudomonas solanacearum
Pseudomonas tabaci
Xanthomonas phaseoli

Right list:
Cercospora kikuchi
Cercospora sojina
Corynespora cassiicola
Fusarium spp.
Peronospora manshurica
Corynebacterium flaccumfaciens
Soybean mosaic virus
Soybean stunt mottling virus
Tobacco ringspot virus
Arabis mosaic virus
Cherry leaf-roll virus
Raspberry ringspot virus
Tomato ringspot virus

Labels: Hilum, Testa, Cotyledons, Radicle

subject of a massive international trade. In this way pathogens are often imported and become established in countries where the conditions for disease development may be more favourable than in the country of origin.

The other way in which man has, often unwittingly, increased the efficiency of pathogen dispersal is by the increased use of vegetative propagation. Potatoes, soft fruits, plantation crops and many ornamentals are regularly propagated by vegetative methods and these provide new opportunities for the colonization of daughter plants, particularly by systemic pathogens. Viruses have been especially favoured by the use of techniques involving grafts, buds, runners, cuttings and tubers.

Man also acts as a vector by carrying disease from crop to crop on his person, on his machines or in foodstuffs and debris (Fig. 4.10). In every respect the threat due to such movement has increased significantly in recent years. Man travels more rapidly and more frequently than ever before. Thus, when after 48 hours he walks into a crop half the world away from his last farm visit, pathogen propagules are more likely to be viable than when the journey lasted six months! Farm machinery has become larger and more complex and it too presents extensive opportunities for transport of propagules from field to field and farm to farm. International commerce and local trade can result in all sorts of plant material being moved from place to place. This material is seldom treated with the respect it deserves as a possible source of disease. As an example of such movement one may cite the importation of timber; the aggressive strain of the Dutch elm disease pathogen responsible for the recent epidemic in Europe was almost certainly introduced in rock elm logs shipped from North America. Unstripped logs have been shown to carry both the fungus and the bark-beetle vectors. Propagules in animal food-stuffs may pass through the gut unharmed and are then introduced into the soil in manure. Corn smut,

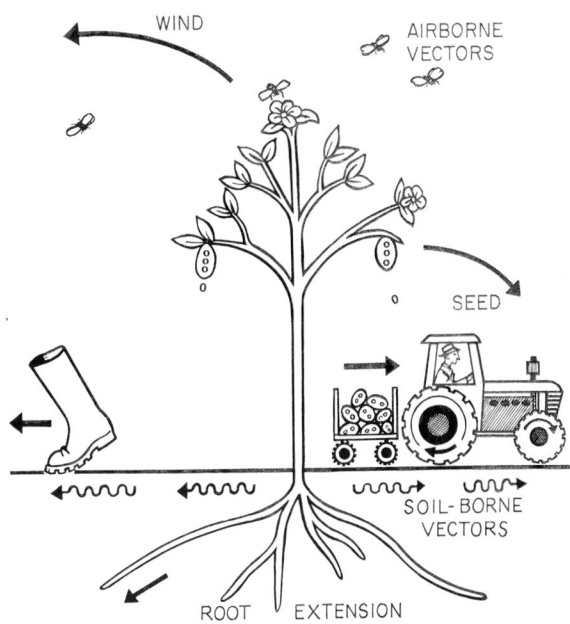

WIND

AIRBORNE
VECTORS

SEED

SOIL-BORNE
VECTORS

ROOT EXTENSION

Figure 4.10 Some mechanisms by which pathogens are dispersed.

Ustilago maydis, is spread in this way as a result of the use of corn cobs as food for hogs in the USA.

PATHOGEN SURVIVAL

Whenever pathogens are not sheltered by a host they face problems of survival in a hostile environment. The extent of this problem for any particular pathogen depends on the length of the period between host and on the relative hostility of the environment. At one extreme, dispersal during epidemic spread may involve only brief periods when spores or other propagules are away from their hosts (see previous section). Other pathogens survive between annual crops planted in successive growing seasons or in rotations when suitable hosts are available only every third, fourth or even fifth year. In the intervening periods, environmental extremes jeopardize the pathogen's chances of survival. Drought, waterlogging and extremes of temperature can all reduce the viability of dormant pathogens. The propagules constituting the pathogen's future inoculum are also subject to microbial antagonism which can severely debilitate or even destroy them.

A summary of the main survival strategies adopted by micro-organisms is given in Fig. 4.11. In some instances, for example when viruses become established in alternative hosts or vectors, or when fungi resort to saprophytism, it may be argued that the term survival is inappropriate. However, plant pathologists who are concerned with potential threats to crops use the term loosely to cover all the possibilities listed in Fig. 4.11.

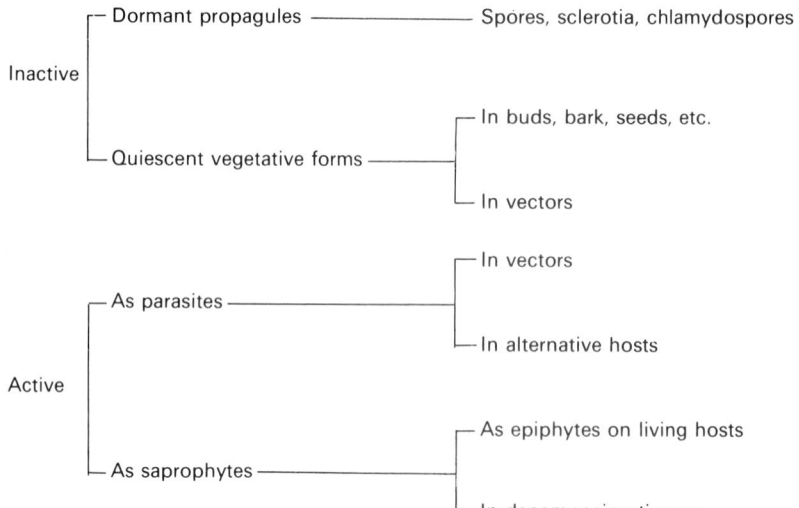

Figure 4.11 Strategies adopted for survival by plant pathogens.

In any discussion of the mechanisms adopted for microbial survival it is natural that attention should focus on the formation and physiology of specialized structures which facilitate long-term perennation. The fungi produce a wide range of survival structures. These vary from single-celled, asexual spores to complex aggregations of hyphae termed SCLEROTIA. Sclerotia and the morphologically simpler CHLAMYDOSPORES are notable

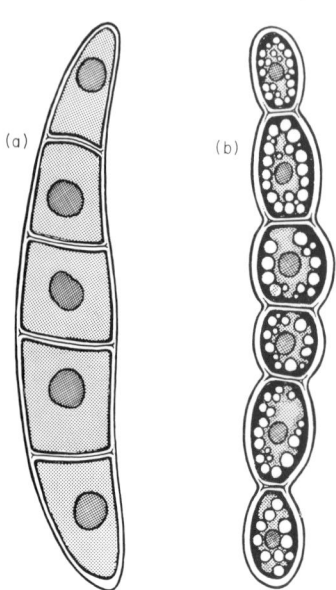

Figure 4.12 Diagrammatic interpretation of electron micrographs showing the transformation of a *Fusarium* macroconidium (a) into a chain of chlamydospores (b) (after Campbell & Griffiths, 1974).

for their longevity and resistance to environmental extremes. Chlamydospores are individual cells with thick, usually pigmented, walls and conspicuous lipid food reserves. They develop directly from hyphal cells or from asexual conidia stranded in habitats where germination cannot immediately occur. Figure 4.12 illustrates the changes which occur when a *Fusarium* macroconidium becomes a chain of chlamydospores. Sclerotia are formed by hyphal branching and aggregation resulting in a mass of similar cells or more highly differentiated structures. These may consist of an outer rind of thick-walled pigmented cells enclosing an inner medulla of thin-walled hyaline cells.

Chlamydospore formation can frequently be induced by the introduction of fungi into soil. This effect has been attributed to the activities of antagonistic micro-organisms, or to alterations in the quality or quantity of nutrients. Sclerotial development appears to be more complex in that it is induced in certain species by mechanical factors, such as damage to hyphae or barriers to extension growth, and in others by nutritional factors, including plant extracts, the carbon/nitrogen ratio, mineral ions and vitamins. Internal morphogenetic factors concerned with the development of an individual colony appear to regulate the formation of sclerotia.

Dormancy

The switch from normal vegetative growth to the formation of propagules or other survival structures may be due to changes in the host or in the environment. In both instances the end result is the development of structures exhibiting DORMANCY, which may be defined as a rest period interrupting development. Ideally, the rest period should be of sufficient duration to give the pathogen a reasonable chance of resuming parasitic activity; this may be achieved by synchronizing the re-activation of the dormant propagules with renewed host activity. Precise systems of control are especially important where the pathogen has a limited ability to search for new hosts. For example, *Plasmodiophora* is only able to swim short distances through soil to the roots of potential hosts. The resting spores of this pathogen are stimulated to germinate by allyl isothiocyanate. This compound is released by crucifer roots and its presence provides an almost fool-proof signal that a host root tip is in the vicinity of the resting spore.

Pathogens which are able to spread extensively following dormancy need only be loosely linked with their host's pattern of activity. *Claviceps* sclerotia respond to environmental factors similar to those which initiate flowering in grasses. This ensures that at anthesis the air spora contains numerous ascospores which infect through the exposed stigmas.

Dormancy is maintained in some propagules by CONSTITUTIVE factors. These are internal controls which must be overcome before propagules can respond to favourable external conditions. Internal checks on germination include permeability barriers and inhibitory substances. Constitutive mechanisms can be overcome by repeated freezing and thawing, exposure to high temperatures, or alternate wetting and drying. Dormancy is also controlled by external or EXOGENOUS factors. These include temperature, water and nutrients. Thus constitutive factors ensure that the propagule remains dormant for a minimum period which is appropriate to the life cycle of the pathogen, whereas exogenous factors are responsible for the synchronization of renewed activity with the susceptible stages in host development.

A diagrammatic representation of these points as they affect fungal sclerotia is given in Fig. 4.13. The initial population is continually declining

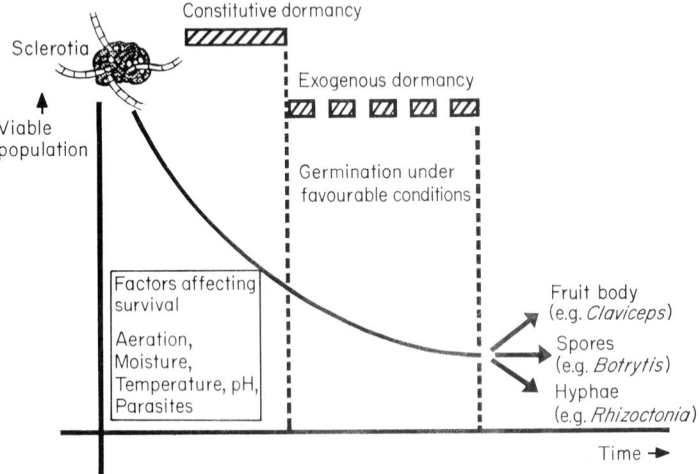

Figure 4.13 Survival and germination of fungal sclerotia under natural conditions.

owing to the operation of a range of lethal factors. At first, germination is prevented by the operation of constitutive factors. Once these are no longer effective there is a requirement for a favourable combination of exogenous factors. When sclerotia germinate they give rise to mycelia or to spores formed on simple structures or in complex fruit bodies.

Interest in germination processes has frequently centred on the possible role played by exogenous nutrients. Some propagules have a requirement for carbohydrates or similar nutrients, whereas others have sufficient endogenous reserves for pre-penetration growth. Much of our knowledge concerning requirements for exogenous nutrients is based on studies of soil-borne pathogens.

Fungistasis

There is more scope for microbial activity in soil than in the aerial environment. Perhaps because of this, a widespread control mechanism exists which restricts the germination of propagules deposited in the soil. This inhibition has been most extensively studied with reference to fungi and has been termed FUNGISTASIS. Despite numerous studies, no fully satisfactory explanation exists as to exactly how fungistasis operates. It is, however, linked with the availability of nutrients, as dormant spores usually germinate if glucose or other nutrients are added to the soil. It is suspected that similar inhibitory effects operate amongst the microbial populations on the aerial surfaces of green plants.

The pathological significance of fungistasis lies in the fact that developing root systems release soluble nutrients from their apices and from the sites of emerging lateral roots. These exudates have been shown experimentally to be sufficiently concentrated to overcome fungistasis. Pathogens then commence active growth and they have only a short distance to travel to the root surface. This response is essentially non-specific in that exudates from both host and non-host plants can stimulate germination.

A more precise requirement for exudates has evolved in some host–pathogen combinations. This ensures that dormancy is only broken when a suitable host is available. A well-documented example has already been mentioned, namely the stimulation of *Plasmodiophora* spores by exudates from brassica roots.

Survival in hosts or vectors

Pathogens also survive in a quiescent vegetative condition amongst host tissues (Fig. 4.11). Survival on or within the host is especially effective in that the pathogen is ideally placed to reinfect newly formed host tissues in the subsequent growing season. The apple mildew pathogen overwinters in dormant buds which form in the autumn. Similarly, *Taphrina* survives in crevices in the bark of peach and almond trees. Plant-pathogenic bacteria are particularly well suited by their size and shape to exploit sheltered niches provided by buds, bark, lenticels and other natural openings. Such niches are a special feature of perennial hosts. Seeds offer special opportunities in this context as they may be both contaminated superficially with propagules and infected internally with pathogens which have temporarily ceased to grow. In spite of their absolute requirement for living hosts, a number of viruses can remain viable in an inactive form for prolonged periods. Viable tobacco mosaic virus has been recovered from dried leaves after these had been stored for 25 years.

Viruses can persist between crops within vectors which are themselves inactive. Two well-established examples of this mode of behaviour involve tobacco rattle virus, which is able to remain infective in dormant nematodes for at least a year, and potato mop-top virus, which can persist for long periods in the resting spores of its fungus vector, the myxomycete *Spongospora*.

Potential pathogens may be present in host tissues for an extended period without causing any visible symptoms. Factors which cause these dormant or LATENT infections to become active include a decrease in the concentration of a toxic substance or a change in the chemistry of the host's tissues. Most examples of latent infections which have been studied to date involve pathogens affecting fruits, where the changes associated with ripening have been shown to stimulate the renewed activity of a quiescent pathogen which initially infected the immature tissues. During ripening of many fruits there are decreases in the level of tannins and phenols, and middle lamellae become more readily degraded by microbial enzymes, resulting in tissue disintegration.

Alternative hosts

Survival can also involve parasitism in alternative hosts or vectors. In some instances the alternative hosts are so described from an anthropocentric viewpoint, i.e. because of the economic importance of the primary host. In other cases the term is used for those species on which the pathogen is less virulent. Whatever approach is adopted, these hosts can bridge the gap between two successive crops of an economically important host. A clear distinction should be drawn between such hosts and the ALTERNATE host species infected during the life cycle of some rust fungi. The relationship between the fungus and its alternate hosts is highly specific and essential for the completion of its life cycle.

Most well-documented examples of the role of alternative hosts involve either viruses or fungi. Cucumber mosaic virus, the cause of severe stunting and yellowing of lettuce, was found in one area to be present in twelve out of fourteen weed species growing in the vicinity of lettuce crops. The virus was not causing any recognizable symptoms in most of these weeds but they would undoubtedly be a source of infection as the aphid vector feeds indiscriminately on numerous hosts. Similarly, an isolate of *Peronospora parasitica* was shown to be capable of attacking 22 crucifer species, in addition to the numerous *Brassica oleracea* cultivars on which it is an economically important pathogen. It was noticeable, however, that on many of these alternative hosts, tissue invasion and sporulation was very restricted. The possible role of these hosts in facilitating survival between successive *Brassica* crops or in aiding epidemic spread is thus questionable.

Survival as saprophytes

Many facultative parasites partially or completely circumvent problems of dormant survival by growing saprophytically. Some of these organisms have very restricted capabilities for non-parasitic growth. A few bacteria and fungi are able to live for long periods on the surfaces of their hosts without penetrating living tissues. These EPIPHYTES are capable of continuing growth even on the limited nutritional resources offered by the host's surface.

More commonly, facultative parasites compete with the populations of free-living decomposers. Their relative success in this competition determines the extent of their saprophytic growth. Success depends partly on the speed of germination and the subsequent growth rate. An ability to degrade a wide range of organic substrates is also essential if the organism is going to be able to grow extensively in a natural habitat such as soil. During growth the organism will have to tolerate the presence of other micro-organisms in its immediate environment, though it may partially restrict the growth of competitors by producing toxic metabolites. All these attributes have been embraced by Garrett in the concept of COMPETITIVE SAPROPHYTIC ABILITY. This concept has proved useful in comparing the behaviour of pathogens which survive as saprophytes. It is also useful in predicting some aspects of parasitic behaviour, as there appears to be a correlation between good competitive saprophytic ability and a necrotrophic life-style in the host.

Two contrasting pathogens will be considered to illustrate these points. *Rhizoctonia solani* attacks juvenile and senescent tissues of a wide range of hosts and once these substrates have been killed and decomposed it is able to grow freely through the soil. *Gaeumannomyces* only infects cereal hosts but it is not restricted to any particular stage in their life cycle. It causes extensive necrosis and overwinters within lesions on persistent host debris. The extent to which *Gaeumannomyces* can survive successfully in this way is dependent upon the prevailing environmental conditions. Warm, moist, well-aerated soils promote the decomposition of roots and straw with a consequent reduction in *Gaeumannomyces* inoculum. The nitrogen regime in the soil is also very important as cereal remains have a very high carbon to nitrogen ratio and this by itself limits the speed of their decomposition.

The fungi utilize by far the most extensive range of survival mechanisms (Table 4.4). Many fungal pathogens adopt several survival strategies which, employed in parallel, considerably increase their chances of successfully enduring unfavourable periods.

In contrast to many bacteria which infect animals, plant-pathogenic bacteria do not form resistant spores. Rather, they have adopted a variety of life styles which ensure the carry-over of their normal vegetative cells, frequently within or amongst host tissues.

Numerous viruses survive within the perennating organs of their hosts. The other principal mode of survival is within vectors or alternative hosts.

Table 4.4 Mechanisms employed by plant pathogens to ensure their survival between crops or during periods unfavourable for parasitic growth. The more + s, the more common the mechanism.

	Fungi	Bacteria	Viruses
Reproductive structures sexual	+ + + + +	−	−
asexual	+ + +	+	−
Vegetative form active	+ + + + +	+	−
inactive	+ + + +	+ + + + +	+ + + +
sclerotia + chlamydospores	+ + + + +	?	−
On alternative hosts	+ +	+	+ + + + +
In vectors	+	+ +	+ + + + +

Longevity

Data concerning the longevity of particular pathogens under natural conditions are often unreliable. Almost all of these data have been gathered in two main ways. An outbreak of disease in an area which has not carried a particular crop for a known number of years has often been taken as proof of the pathogen's ability to survive through the intervening period. Clearly, such information is of practical significance but it is usually impossible to relate it to the survival of particular propagules, such as spores or sclerotia. Information on the survival of specific structures may only be obtained from experiments. It requires little imagination to see the practical difficulties attending studies of this sort, which can last for several decades (Fig. 4.14). These experiments involve declining populations (Fig. 4.13) and

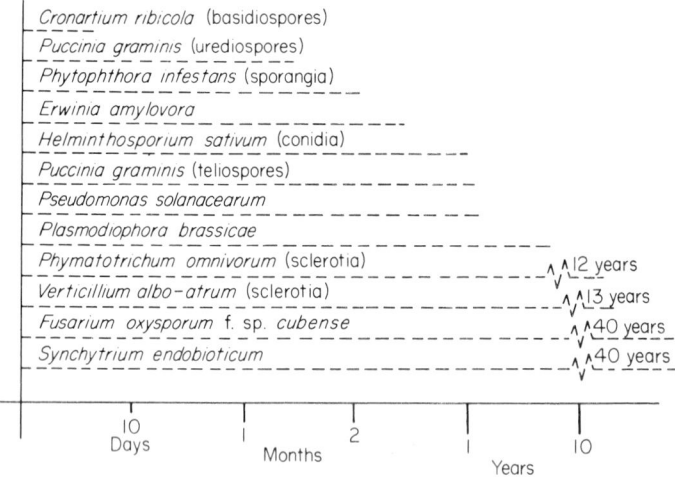

Figure 4.14 Survival periods recorded for some pathogens in the field.

increasingly sensitive sampling techniques may be required to detect smaller and smaller numbers of viable spores. It should also be borne in mind that laboratory studies do not necessarily demonstrate the fate of propagules either in natural soils or in the upper atmosphere. Despite these difficulties it is clear that there are substantial variations in the longevity of different pathogens.

FURTHER READING

General texts

DIENER T.O. (1979) *Viroids and Viroid Diseases.* John Wiley & Sons, London.
    A most readable account by a pioneer in the field.
GIBBS A. & HARRISON B.D. (1979) *Plant Virology : the Principles.* Edward Arnold, London.
    An attractive book on a subject which is neglected by many plant pathologists.

GARRETT S.D. (1970) *Pathogenic Root-infecting Fungi.* Cambridge University Press, Cambridge.

A classic text which emphasises the ecological relationships between soil-borne pathogens and their hosts.

GREGORY P.H. (1973) *Microbiology of the Atmosphere.* Leonard Hill, Aylesbury.

The standard work on aerobiology with many references to the behaviour of pathogens in this environment.

INGOLD C.T. (1971) *Fungal Spores.* Clarendon Press, Oxford.

Records the remarkable diversity of fungal spores and their dispersal mechanisms.

SMITH K.M. (1977) *Plant Viruses.* Chapman & Hall, London.

A concise introduction to plant virology.

Reviews and original papers

COLEY-SMITH J.R. & COOKE R.C. (1971) Survival and germination of fungal sclerotia. *Annual Review of Phytopathology* **9**, 65–92.

GROSS H.J. *et al.* (1978) Nucleotide sequence and secondary structure of potato spindle tuber viroid. *Nature* (London) **273**, 203–8.

HARRISON B.D. (1981) Plant virus ecology: ingredients, interactions and environmental influences. *Annals of Applied Biology* **99**, 195–209.

MAAS W.K. (1981) Genetics of bacterial virulence. *Symposium of the Society of General Microbiology* **31**, 341–360.

MARKHAM P.G. & TOWNSEND R. (1981) Spiroplasmas. *Science Progress Oxford* **67**, 43–68.

NIENHAUS F. & SIKORA R.A. (1979) Mycoplasmas, spiroplasmas and rickettsia-like organisms as plant pathogens. *Annual Review of Phytopathology* **17**, 37–58.

SCHUSTER M.L. & COYNE D.P. (1974) Survival mechanisms of phytopathogenic bacteria. *Annual Review of Phytopathology* **12**, 199–221.

SMITH H. (1978) The determinants of microbial pathogenicity. In *Essays in Microbiology* (eds Norris J.R. & Richmond M.H.), Chapter 13. John Wiley & Sons, Chichester.

5 Infection and colonization

"Whenever the little seeds of rust come to rest upon the same stalk, finding some open mouths of the exhaling vessels, there they enchase their minute radical fibers, and there they infiltrate in such a manner, that they graft into the tender and delicate arteries peculiar to the plant."

G. TARGIONI-TOZZETTI (1712–1783)

Pathogens establish physiological contact with their hosts in a number of ways. Some penetrate through the intact surface covering of the plant. Others enter through natural openings where the external protective layers are especially thin or even completely absent. The most important such route, at least in numerical terms, is through the stomata, but other lines of weakness exploited by pathogens include glands, hydathodes, lenticels, nectaries and root tips. Still other pathogens enter the host via wounds. Such wounds often result from physical or chemical damage or from the activities of animal pests. Wounds can also be self-inflicted, for instance by the abscission of leaves or during the emergence of lateral roots.

An important distinction may thus be drawn between pathogens which enter directly through their host's protective barriers, and others which bypass these defences. One major group of pathogens, the viruses, is almost entirely dependent upon wounds to gain entry to the host. This follows from their inability to grow outside living cells.

THE INFECTION COURT

Let us assume that a pathogen has been successfully dispersed or has grown into contact with a potential host plant. Subsequent development of the surface of the host, penetration into the host and the very early stages of establishment within host tissues comprise the process of INFECTION. This stage in the pathogen's life cycle ends when the organism becomes dependent on the host for nutrients at which point it begins to COLONIZE tissues around the initial site of infection.

The initial site of contact between the pathogen and the surface of the host is described as the INFECTION COURT. In any discussion of host penetration it is important to distinguish at the outset between the aerial and subterranean surfaces of the plant. In one respect the problems confronting

60

airborne and soil-borne pathogens are similar, in that both must breach the host's outer defensive layers, but there are major differences between the two environments. Soil exerts a buffering effect against extremes of temperature, water and other environmental fluctuations. A propagule landing on an aerial plant surface is exposed to such hazards as ultraviolet light and rapid desiccation. In addition, airborne pathogens typically make contact with their host in the form of wind-borne or splash-dispersed propagules, while soil organisms often grow vegetatively towards roots.

The leaf and root surfaces of plants are termed the PHYLLOPLANE and the RHIZOPLANE respectively. The allied terms phyllosphere and rhizosphere describe the habitats adjacent to these surfaces. In recent years a great deal has been learned regarding the influence of physical, chemical and biological factors on pathogen behaviour in these two infection courts. Factors influencing the germination of fungal spores are of special significance and include humidity, temperature, light, duration of surface wetness, pH, exogenous nutrients and inhibitors, and the propagules and cells of other microbes. Exudates from leaves and roots contain numerous chemicals such as sugars, amino acids, mineral salts, phenols and alkaloids; any of these may stimulate or inhibit germination and/or growth of pathogens. Root exudates are particularly significant in determining the behaviour of soil fungi, such as some species of *Phytophthora*, which produce motile zoospores. These are chemotactically attracted to the elongating zone of host roots where they encyst prior to entry. Zoospores are reported to exhibit chemotaxis towards the roots of both host and non-host species, though specificity has been demonstrated for some species of *Phytophthora* toward their particular hosts. The initial phases of development on the host surface would seem to represent an especially vulnerable stage in the life cycle of fungal pathogens, as witnessed by the efficacy of protectant fungicides in the control of many diseases.

The principal components of the aerial surfaces of herbaceous plants are summarized in Fig. 5.1. In practice, there are considerable physical and chemical differences in the outer layers of various plant species, and even

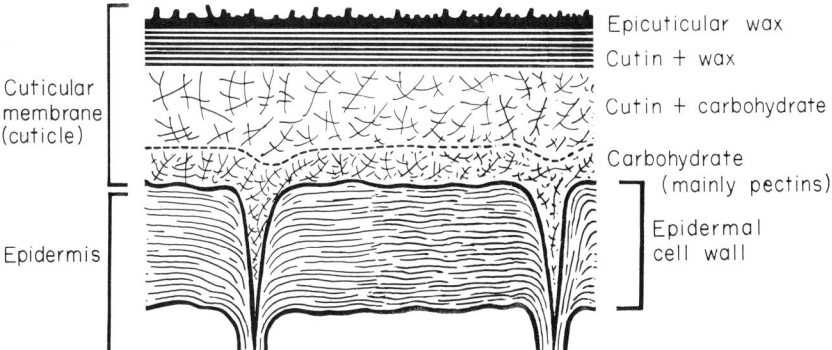

Figure 5.1   The external layers bounding herbaceous plant organs (after Jeffree, Baker & Holloway, 1976).

between different parts of the same plant. Thus the cuticle may vary in chemical composition and thickness on leaves, flowers and fruits. Variations are also found in different regions of the same organ, for example between the abaxial and adaxial surfaces of leaves. Other factors influencing the structure and composition of external layers include the conditions under which the plant has grown, and the developmental stage that the plant has reached. Seedling tissues are particularly prone to infection by opportunist pathogens, such as the 'damping off' fungus *Pythium*, whereas mature plants are seldom attacked. It seems reasonable to suppose that a critical factor here is the relative ease with which the pathogen can penetrate the cuticle and epidermal layers in the yount plant.

The outer cell walls of primary roots are in some species impregnated with lipid materials, including suberin and cutin. These materials can form a definite membrane comparable with the leaf cuticle, but the use of the term cuticle to describe this root covering is not accepted by some scientists. There is also some doubt as to whether such protective layers are present in the physiologically active apical region of the root. The root hair zone is especially vulnerable to pathogens, as it is in intimate contact with a large volume of soil. The necessity for efficient water and nutrient uptake by the root hairs means that mechanical barriers, which would perhaps deter pathogens, are absent.

There are even greater differences between the surfaces of herbaceous tissues and the stems and roots of woody perennials. Periderm, commonly termed bark, is formed following secondary thickening and the accompanying increase in girth of the organs. It comprises three layers with the outermost being composed of dead cork cells which have suberized cell walls. Suberin is a complex material containing mixtures of hydroxy acids and it is very resistant to microbial decay. This substance, together with lignin and cellulose in the cork cell walls and resins in their lumina, ensures that bark is virtually impregnable to invasion by micro-organisms. Similar protective layers are also formed over abscission wounds and other damaged areas.

DIRECT PENETRATION

As shown in Fig. 5.1, direct penetration of herbaceous tissues requires that a pathogen must enter through layers of wax, cutin, pectin and a network of cellulose fibrils impregnated with other wall polymers before making contact with living protoplasm. This would seem to be a formidable problem. Nevertheless, many fungal pathogens are able to enter their hosts in this way. Specialized biotrophs, such as the rusts and the downy and powdery mildews, often gain access by growing down into the epidermis, but direct penetration is by no means restricted to this type of pathogen. Even relatively non-specific pathogens, such as *Botrytis*, can in suitable circumstances enter hosts directly by penetration through the cuticle.

62

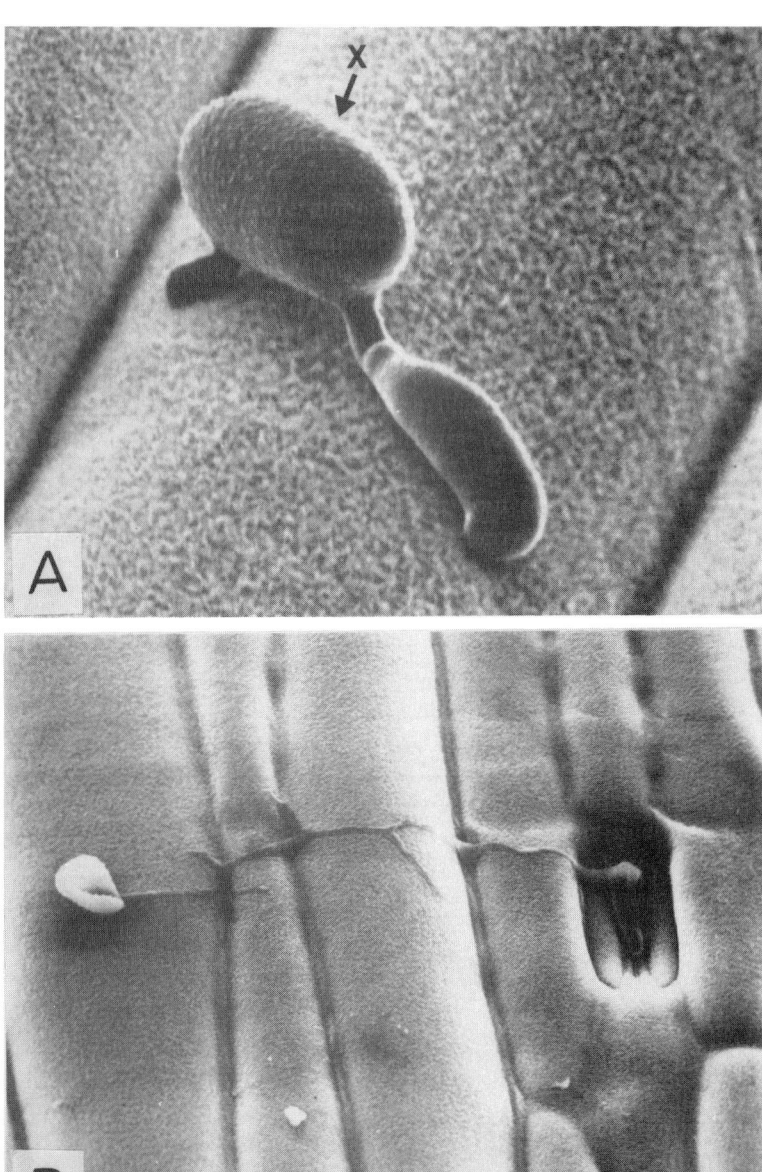

Figure 5.2 Scanning electron micrographs of (A) *Erysiphe graminis* on barley (× 1900) and (B) *Puccinia graminis* on wheat (× 530). The *Erysiphe* conidium (X) has produced a short germ tube and then an appressorium over an epidermal cell. The *Puccinia* germ tube has grown to a stoma through which it then penetrates. (A) reproduced by courtesy of I.C.I., Plant Protection Division.

Direct penetration of the host by fungi is frequently associated with the development of hyphal modifications known collectively as infection structures. Some examples are shown in Fig. 5.2. Once the spore has germinated there follows a period of growth in which the germ tube extends over the leaf surface. This growth may appear to be random but some evidence points to the possibility that the germ tube is 'searching' for a favourable site for penetration. The length of germ tube developed varies but eventually extension growth ceases and the tip of the hypha swells to form an APPRESSORIUM. This spherical or ovoid structure increases the area of contact and attachment between the fungus and the host surface. Penetration then takes place by the downward growth of a thin hyphal thread or infection peg formed on the lower surface of the appressorium where it adheres to the host. There is still debate as to the actual mechanics of penetration. Early workers showed that many fungi will successfully penetrate artificial materials such as gold leaf, suggesting that the process is entirely mechanical. However, recent scanning and transmission electron microscope studies have suggested that some pathogens actually degrade cutin, cellulose and pectin during penetration. Differential staining techniques have revealed localized dissolution of cuticle and cell wall around infection pegs, implicating the action of hydrolytic enzymes in penetration by fungi..

Much of the emphasis in these studies has been on penetration through the cuticle, and several fungal pathogens have been shown to produce extracellular esterase enzymes which have the potential to degrade cutin. Using ^{14}C-labelled cutin, such breakdown has been demonstrated for some of these enzymes, which can then be described as cutinases. In an elegant series of immunological experiments, *Fusarium solani* f.sp. *pisi* has been found to produce cutinase at the site of infection. Penetration was, however, subsequently halted by the application of an antiserum prepared from the cutinase, which suggested that this enzyme plays a vital role in the entry of the pathogen into its host [see Further Reading—Maiti & Kolattukudy (1979) and review by MacNamara & Dickinson (1981)].

Broadly speaking, the events taking place during spore germination, germ-tube growth and penetration are similar in a wide variety of fungal pathogens. Nevertheless, even closely related fungi exhibit certain idiosyncrasies in their penetration behaviour. Figure 5.3 compares the entry of the downy mildew fungi *Peronospora parasitica* and *Bremia lactucae* into their respective hosts, cabbage and lettuce. *Peronospora* typically penetrates through the anticlinal walls between epidermal cells. *Bremia* enters directly into an epidermal cell through its periclinal wall and then progresses into the underlying tissues. An indication of the time that these processes take is also given in this figure.

An ability to form appressoria does not mean that the pathogen always enters by direct penetration. Many rust species and *Phytophthora infestans* enter their hosts both directly and through stomata. Similar appressoria and infection hyphae are formed in both situations.

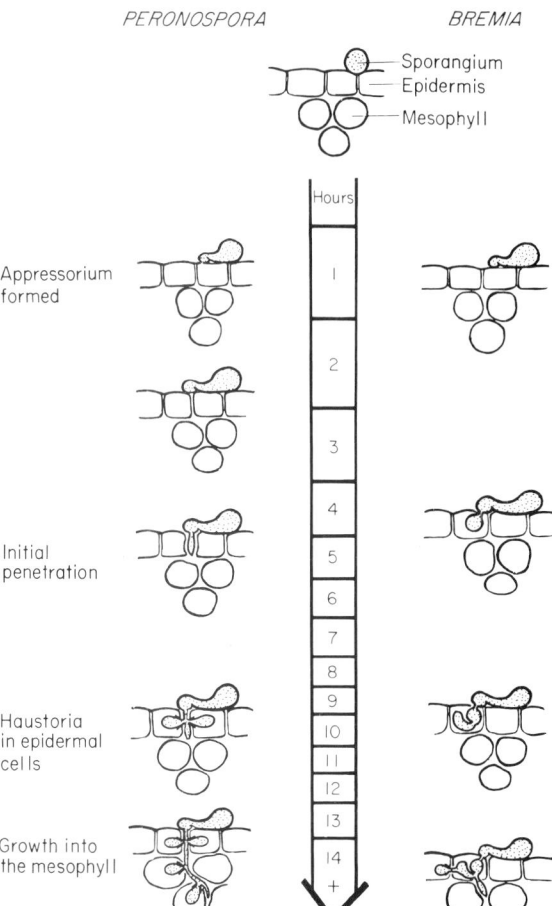

Figure 5.3 Comparison between infection of cabbage by *Peronospora parasitica* and lettuce by *Bremia lactucae*. The relative time scale shown may be altered by environmental conditions, particularly temperature.

Root-infecting fungi also form infection structures, though these seem to be generally more complex than those produced by fungi attacking aerial tissues. Some isolates of *Gaeumannomyces* produce appressoria which in this fungus take the form of short side branches from runner hyphae, beneath which narrow penetration hyphae enter the root cortex. These and more complex pseudoparenchymatous structures are apparently only formed on resistant tissues, as non-resistant tissues can be penetrated directly from the runner hyphae. *Rhizoctonia solani*, a versatile pathogen attacking a wide variety of hosts, forms both lobed appressoria and more complex aggregations of short, branched hyphae, called infection cushions (Fig. 5.4). The former tend to be produced on aerial tissues and the latter on roots and other subterranean organs. Multiple infection hyphae are produced from the inner surface of infection cushions and a rather similar process occurs in the

65

tree pathogen *Armillaria mellea*. When the rhizomorphs of this fungus encounter a suitable host the concerted action of the numerous constituent hyphae is often sufficient to penetrate intact periderm.

The root hairs are particularly vulnerable to invasion by pathogens. *Plasmodiophora brassicae* enters root hairs at an early stage in its life cycle, before subsequent re-infection and proliferation in cortical cells. The mode of entry of *Plasmodiophora* appears to be unique. Zoospores of the pathogen

Club root
in brassica
Myxomycota

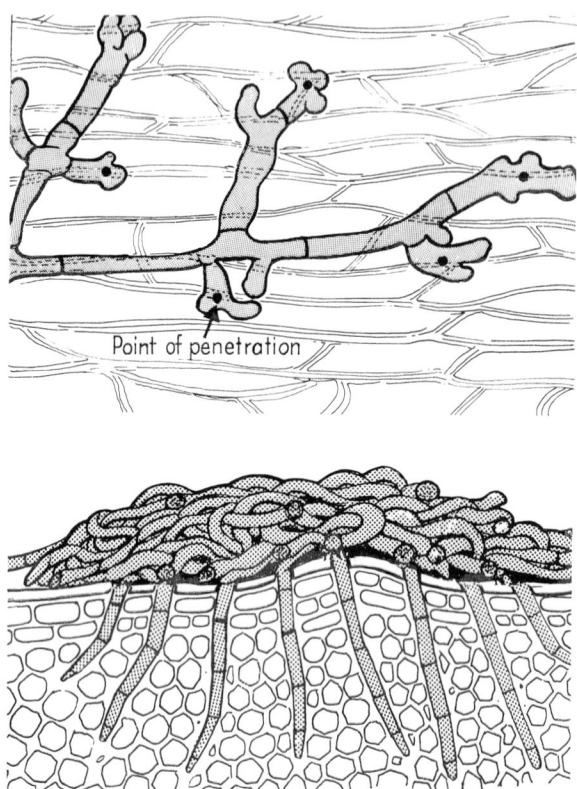

Point of penetration

Figure 5.4 Top: *Rhizoctonia* hyphae showing the short irregular side branch appressoria formed on root surfaces.
Bottom: a section through *Rhizoctonia* infection cushion showing the numerous penetration pegs. (Both after Christou, 1962.)

encyst on the wall of a root hair. A fine puncture is made in the host cell wall and the contents of the spore are rapidly injected through this into the hair cell (Fig. 5.5). The puncture is produced when a bullet-shaped structure is suddenly forced from within the cyst through the wall into the interior of the root hair. This is a particularly dramatic example of mechanical penetration, the actual infection process taking only about one second.

66

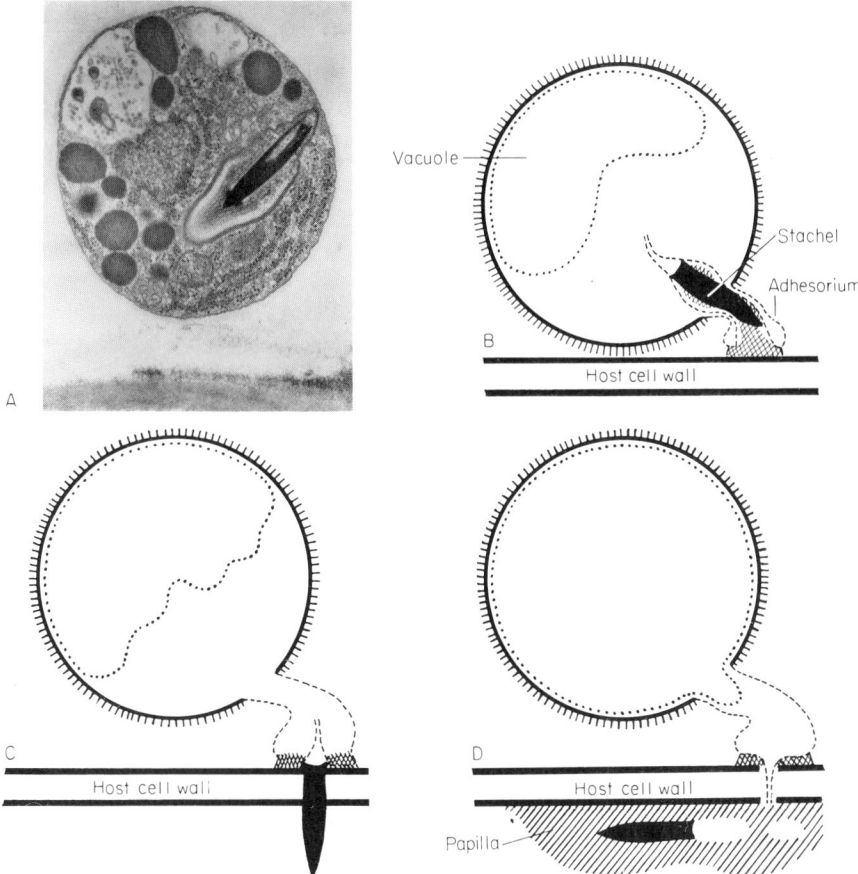

Figure 5.5 (A) Electronmicrograph section of a *Plasmodiophora brassicae* zoospore encysted on a root hair, showing bullet-like stachel (× 29 500). (B–D) diagrammatic summary of the penetration of a root hair; (B) vacuole enlarges and small adhesorium appears; (C) stachel punctures host wall; (D) penetration has occurred and the host protoplast has deposited a papilla at the penetration site. (From Williams *et al.*, 1973.)

PENETRATION THROUGH NATURAL OPENINGS

The surface layers of field-grown plants are rarely intact, but even if they were, there are still a number of natural openings through which microbes can enter. The most important of these are stomata, via which many pathogens enter their hosts. Stomatal morphology may in fact determine whether infection takes place, as in citrus fruits where the conformation of the cuticle around the stoma either prevents or allows the passage of water droplets containing the bacterial pathogen *Pseudomonas citri*. Stomata are also the main site of entry of several important fungal pathogens. When a rust spore germinates on a cereal leaf the germ tube grows at right angles to the long axis of the leaf. This precise orientation of growth is an example of THIGMOTROPISM. It is probably organized through the recognition by the hyphae of the regular pattern formed by the crystals of epicuticular wax.

67

The orientation of the hyphae across the long axis of the epidermal cells ensures that they will sooner or later encounter a stoma, as these occur in longitudinal rows (Fig. 5.2).

Several downy mildew pathogens, including *Pseudoperonospora* on hops and *Plasmopara* on vines, produce sporangia which germinate on their host's leaves forming several motile zoospores. These zoospores are attracted to stomata where they encyst in a suitable position for their germ tubes to grow immediately between the guard cells (Fig. 5.6). *Pseudoperonospora*

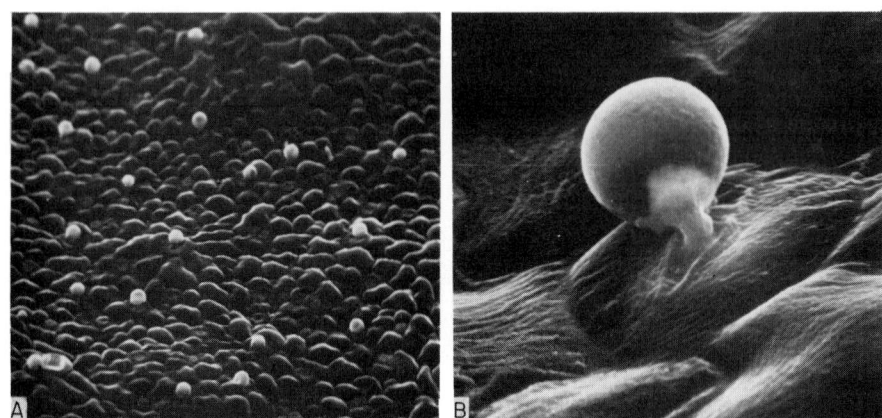

Figure 5.6 *Pseudoperonospora* zoospores settle and encyst on hop stomata (A), where they then germinate and penetrate the leaf via the stomatal cavity (B) (from Royle, 1976).

zoospores are attracted to open stomata but not to closed stomata. This attraction is based in part on their recognition of the morphology of the open apertures and partly on a chemical stimulus which appears to be connected with gaseous photosynthetic metabolites.

It should be recognized that entry through the stomatal aperture does not mean that the pathogen has breached all the host's defences. The substomatal cavity is bounded by cuticle, though this appears to be substantially thinner than that on exposed leaf surfaces. Hence the pathogen must penetrate through a second barrier to gain access to the host's tissues, though it is probably aided in this task by the high water content in the substomatal cavity. A further aspect of penetration through stomata concerns the possible role played by saprophytic organisms. Extensive development of such organisms in the substomatal cavity, encouraged no doubt by the same factors which favour the growth of pathogens, may create further obstacles which are not encountered by pathogens able to penetrate directly through the plant's surface defences.

Lenticels occur in bark on woody stems and on secondarily thickened roots. These loosely packed openings in the periderm are also abundant on potato tubers, where they provide suitable sites for the entry of a number of micro-organisms, especially *Phytophthora infestans* and *Streptomyces scabies*. Penetration through intact surfaces which have especially thin mechanical

68

barriers also occurs at glands and nectaries. *Erwinia amylovora*, the bacterium responsible for the destructive fireblight disease of pears and apples, enters through nectaries at the base of flowers. In this case, the sugary secretions of nectar which accumulate outside these glands when diluted by rain provide a favourable medium for multiplication of the pathogen prior to penetration. Fireblight infections are also prevalent after severe thunderstorms, which suggests that the bacterium takes advantage of minor wounds caused by heavy rainstorms.

PENETRATION THROUGH WOUNDS

For many pathogens, wounds are the most frequent or only avenue of entry. Wounds are caused by man and his machines, as well as by natural agencies, including wind, extremes of temperature and light, and by pests. The external barriers of the host may also be broken temporarily as a natural consequence of growth and development.

Many agricultural and horticultural practices involve accidental or even deliberate wounding. Grafting, pruning and various cultivation practices may inadvertently spread pathogens through a crop or create wounds which can be exploited by opportunist fungi and bacteria. The increased use of mechanical harvesting has also increased the incidence of wounding of plant produce. Post-harvest rots of apples (caused by *Penicillium expansum*) and citrus fruits (which are parasitized by *Penicillium digitatum* and *P. italicum*) are only important if the fruits are bruised during harvesting, packing or transport. Many important forest pathogens also enter through wounds. *Heterobasidion annosum*, which is a destructive pathogen of conifers, normally colonizes wounds caused by high winds, snow or other natural agencies. It has become a particularly damaging pathogen in plantations where it takes advantage of the stumps left after felling as sites for entry (see Chapter 10).

Leaf abscission provides opportunities for infection, as does any other point in the life cycle at which parts of the plant are detached. *Nectria galligena*, which causes apple canker, enters woody twigs through the vascular bundles which are exposed at leaf fall and in this way it avoids the problem of penetrating the effective barrier which is posed by the bark. The exposed vascular bundles in the leaf scar are, however, soon sealed off by the development of a new cork layer and hence the pathogen must take immediate advantage of the infection courts created at leaf fall. Lateral roots emerge by literally breaking through the cortex of the parent root. The disruption of cortical cells results in the release into the soil of a solution rich in carbohydrates and amino acids. This solution attracts zoospores of fungi, such as *Phytophthora*, which then encyst on and penetrate into the damaged cortical tissues.

Soft-rot pathogens of potatoes commonly enter tubers through the scar left during separation of the tuber from the parent stolon. Senescent tissues which remain attached to otherwise healthy plants facilitate the invasion of

Whole plant
from other damaged
areas of the
plant.

adjoining healthy tissues by opportunist pathogens. *Botrytis* colonizes healthy lettuce leaves, and even stems, by vegetative growth from senescent leaves or damaged leaf margins. The same fungus can become established on the senescing remains of tomato flowers and from here it invades the developing fruit causing a blossom end rot disease.

Lesions caused by pathogens themselves may serve as avenues of entry for other pathogens. In these instances the host is initially infected by a pathogen which may or may not itself cause very serious damage. This pathogen, however, paves the way for more aggressive organisms. Potato late blight symptoms cn tubers are manifest as dry sunken lesions which under most conditions spread only slowly through the flesh. Secondary infections of these lesions by soft-rot bacteria, such as *Erwinia carotovora*, can transform the whole tuber into a putrescent mass within a few days.

We have already seen that many pests are also important vectors for plant pathogens. The Dutch elm fungus, *Ceratocystis ulmi*, is introduced directly into sap wood by its vector, the bark beetle. In this example the feeding tunnels not only breach the external protective layers of bark but also provide direct access to the vascular tissues in which the fungus can flourish. An even more elegant means of entry is provided by the aphid vectors of many viruses. The aphid stylet literally injects the virus into the sieve cells of the host; from here the virus can spread freely through the phloem. Soil-borne viruses are often introduced via wounds caused by nematodes or fungal pathogens. The wide range of vectors exploited by viruses is paralleled by a similar variety of infection routes. As was discussed earlier, some viruses, for example bean mosaic virus, may be transmitted to the ovules of healthy plants through infected pollen. This is a particularly interesting case as the virus takes advantage of a normal event in the life cycle of the host. However, just as with virus transmission through seed, it is not at all clear how common or important are the 'wounds' associated with the entry of the pollen tube in the spread of viruses under natural conditions.

DEVELOPMENT FOLLOWING INFECTION

Following penetration, there are wide variations in the subsequent pattern of colonization of host tissues. The extent to which pathogens grow within their hosts is related to the nature of the parasitic relationship between the two partners. Where the growth of the pathogen is superficial (i.e. ectotrophic), as with the powdery mildews, colonization proceeds no further than the epidermal cells (see Fig. 10.6). Mycelial development of the apple scab fungus is restricted to the subcuticular layers of the leaf and fruit, at least until the onset of general tissue senescence. More extensive invasion of epidermal and mesophyll layers then takes place, leading to the formation of over-wintering stromata. Other differences in the pattern of host colonization are determined by host reactions, rather than by the life style of the invading pathogen.

Ascomycete
Erysiphe
graminis

70

The severity of disease in an affected plant is usually related to the extent of pathogen invasion. Where the pathogen is localized through a host defence reaction the symptoms are confined to a small area or reduced to an insignificant level. There are, however, certain exceptions to this rule. For instance, a localized pathogen may disrupt an essential physiological function, such as water transport, or produce a diffusible toxin which can act at a distance from the lesion itself. In an extreme example of this type of behaviour, the pathogen causing choke disease of grasses, *Epichloe typhina*, is restricted to a short section of leaf sheath tissue but its growth in this strategic position prevents the emergence of the flowering axis and hence its effect on the life cycle of the host are dramatic.

SYSTEMIC infections, in which the pathogen spreads throughout the entire plant body, are unusual. Pathogens usually spread within one or a few organs (Fig. 5.7). Some pathogens are specific to one or a few tissues; the apple scab fungus grows almost exclusively in the subcuticular layer of the leaf and fruit (see Fig. 10.2), while the vascular wilt pathogens and the mycoplasmas are confined to the xylem and phloem respectively. There appears to be a correlation between the mode of nutrition of pathogens and

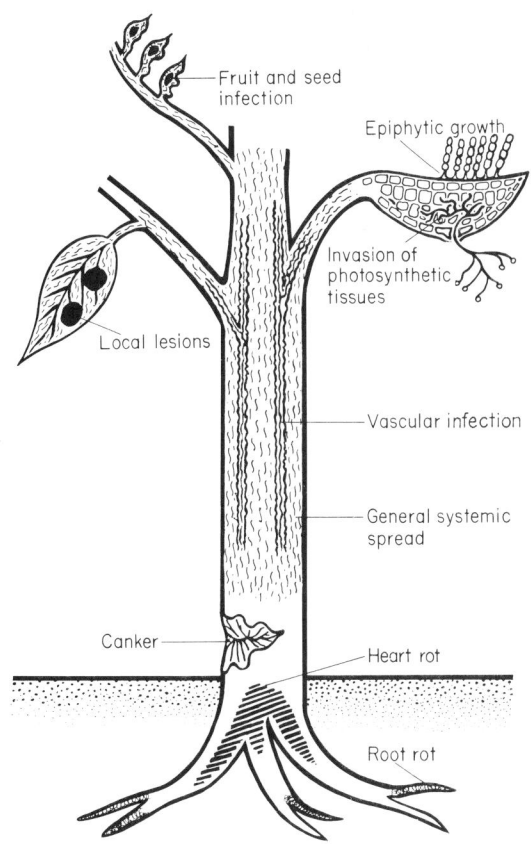

Figure 5.7 Some patterns of pathogenic invasion of plant tissues.

their specialization to different types of host tissue. In other words, the less specialized necrotrophic pathogens tend to spread indiscriminately through plant organs, while biotrophs, in keeping with their more benign form of parasitism, grow selectively within certain well-defined tissues of the host plant.

Colonization by fungi

It may be argued that the most important feature distinguishing different groups of pathogens is not their preference for particular tissues but rather the actual method they employ to colonize their hosts. Let us compare two fungal pathogens with very different life styles.

Damping-off diseases are caused by a number of pathogens, amongst which several species of *Pythium* are especially notable as causal agents of both pre- and postemergence damping-off syndromes in a wide variety of hosts. In both instances, these fungi usually encounter their host following growth through the soil, though the likelihood of the fungus contacting a potential host is probably increased by the chemotropic effects of exudates released by the germinating seed or developing seedling. Entry into the seed may be through cracks in the swollen seed coat, and further growth into the embryo involves a combination of mechanical pressure and enzyme action. The fungus passes from cell lumen to cell lumen producing pectolytic enzymes to dissolve the middle lamellae and proteolytic enzymes to degrade the host's protoplasm. The seed is thus rapidly killed. If host–pathogen contact does not occur until after germination, the fungus usually penetrates the hypocotyl at soil level. Colonization of the epidermis, the cortex and even the vascular tissues then proceeds as in the seed. The seedling falls over, due to the collapse of the supportive tissues in the cortex, and it is finally killed. Attempts by these pathogens to invade older plants are either completely unsuccessful or result in minor lesions which have a relatively unimportant impact on host development. This is due to the increase in cell wall thickness and lignification and to a change in the middle lamellae which makes them more resistant to dissolution by fungal enzymes. In this disease, complex host defences develop over a period of time and although the pathogen can completely destroy juvenile plants it becomes progressively less successful as the host plant matures. Other relatively unspecialized pathogens which attack mature plants are prevented from spreading extensively through their host by the development of histological defence reactions. For instance, *Rhizoctonia solani* may be effectively sealed off in a potato tuber by means of an impregnable cork layer formed in response to infection.

The black stem rust fungus, *Puccinia graminis* f.sp. *tritici*, affects two alternate hosts, wheat and barberry, during its life cycle. Economically important epidemics on wheat are caused by urediospores. These germinate on

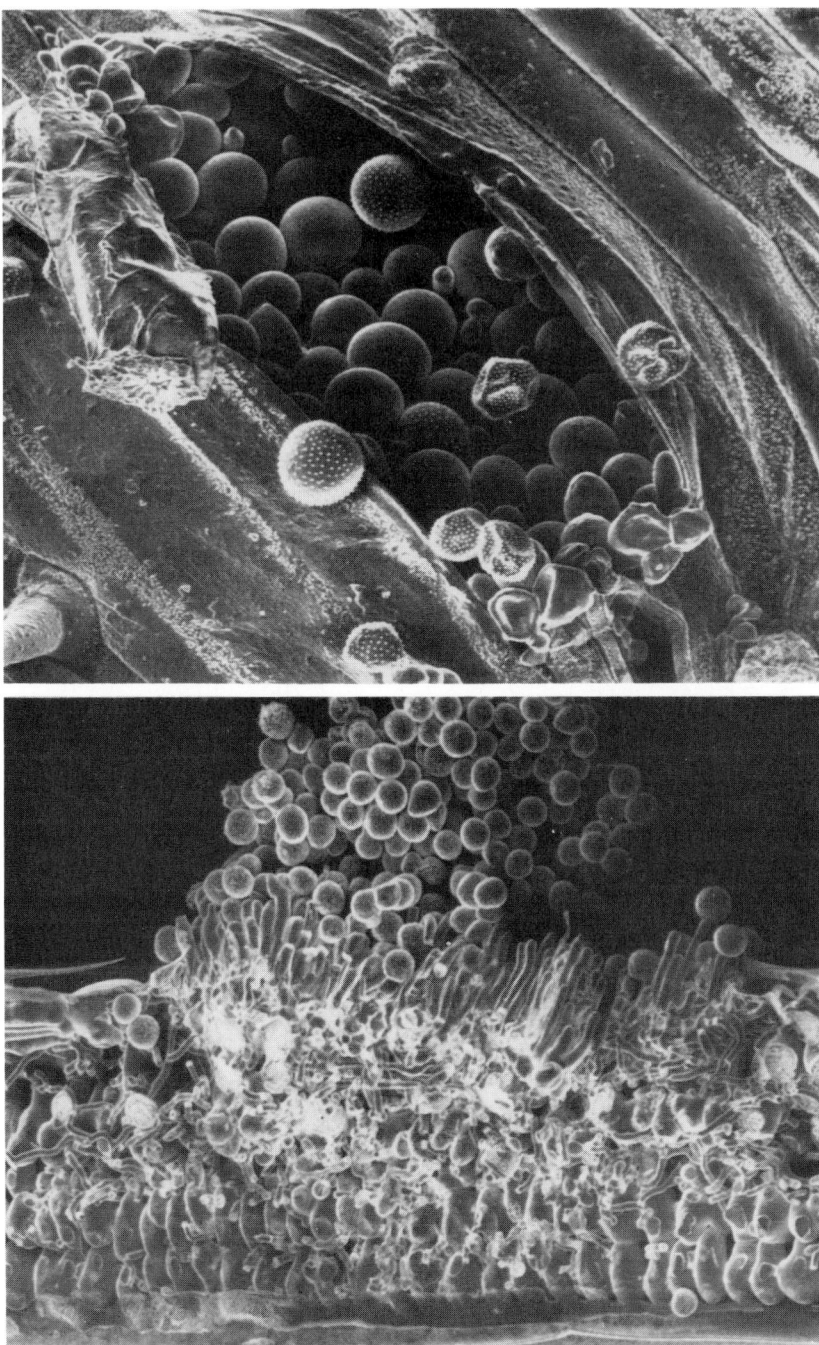

Figure 5.8 Scanning electron micrographs of wheat rust urediospore pustules. In the upper photograph a yellow stripe rust pustule is just breaking through the host epidermis. In the lower photograph a mature brown rust pustule is seen in section. (Photographs by courtesy of ICI Plant Protection Division.)

leaves and the germ tube enters through a stoma (Fig. 5.2). The fungus then grows intercellularly in the leaf mesophyll tissue, sending club-shaped haustoria into adjacent host cells. The mycelium produced from a single uredio-spore does not invade the entire leaf; instead, it forms a relatively small colony within the photosynthetic tissue. A mat of fungal hyphae differentiates just below the host epidermis which is then torn open to reveal the characteristic uredial pustule (as in other cereal rusts, see Fig. 5.8). The whole process from germination to spore production takes about eight days at field temperatures, and at no stage is there massive breakdown of infected tissues. The host is only severely damaged when many separate colonies of the pathogen develop simultaneously on leaves, stems or glumes.

Amongst those micro-organisms which are specific to particular host tissues, the vascular wilt pathogens have a particularly interesting mode of spread within the host (Fig. 7.13). Fungi such as *Fusarium oxysporum* and *Verticillium albo-atrum* enter through the cortex in the apical region of the root. The endodermis is often an effective barrier to pathogens but as it is not fully developed in this region it is easily breached and the fungi then enter the xylem elements. Further spread within the living host is restricted to this tissue. Hyphae grow through the xylem and pass from cell to cell via pit pairs. In addition, long-distance movement is accomplished by the production of microconidia which are carried in the transpiration stream. This mode of spread is much more rapid than would be possible by mycelial growth; the Panama disease wilt pathogen, *Fusarium oxysporum* f.sp. *cubense*, can migrate from the bottom to the top of an eight-metre-tall banana tree in less than two weeks. Because xylem tissues ramify throughout the plant, wilt pathogens can migrate into every part of their host. Thus, although they are tissue specific these pathogens can become virtually systemic. The Dutch elm fungus usually enters its host through beetle feeding wounds on young branches. Both beetle vectors commonly feed in crotches, with *Hylurgopinus* choosing stems 2–12 cm in diameter and *Scolytus* preferring younger twigs. Subsequent spread within the xylem is so extensive that suckers and neighbouring trees can become infected via natural root grafts. There is something of a paradox here in that spread from shoot to root is counter to the usual transpiration stream.

Only a few fungi, notably the smuts, are truly systemic in their hosts. *Ustilago nuda*, causing loose smut of barley, occurs as a dormant mycelium in the cotyledon of infected grain. During germination of the seed the pathogen also resumes activity and grows intercellularly within the young seedling. As the plant matures the pathogen keeps pace just behind the apical meristem, and eventually invades the developing flower head to form a mass of black teliospores in place of the grain. The older mycelium in the stem may break down as the host matures, but it often persists in the nodes. One interesting feature of smut diseases is that visible symptoms are not obviously manifest until the pathogen sporulates. Infected plants may, however, be slightly taller than normal.

Colonization by bacteria

The morphology of bacterial cells limits their capacity for widespread growth through compact tissues. Thus, spread within the host is often accomplished by maceration of tissues or by the exploitation of natural channels.

For example, the bacterium *Erwinia carotovora* causes a common storage soft-rot of potato tubers (see Fig. 8.7). It is unable to pass through intact periderm and therefore gains entry via lenticels or wounds including, as noted above, those caused by other pathogens. Once inside the tuber, the bacterium spreads rapidly through the parenchyma giving rise to a soft, slimy, putrid lesion and under favourable conditions it can completely destroy the tuber. At all stages of colonization the bacterium occupies intercellular spaces (Fig. 5.9), and its spread is facilitated by the production of pectolytic enzymes which degrade middle lamellae and thus macerate the host tissues. Subsequently, tuber cells are rapidly killed by the pathogen. However, under aerobic storage conditions at low relative humidities, the rate of invasion is slower and the bacterium may be localized by a black oxidation zone. This zone is partly an anatomical barrier, involving the deposition of suberin in tuber cell walls, and partly a chemical barrier, consisting of oxidized polyphenols. Similar histological defence reactions are important in restricting spread of many other relatively unspecialized pathogens within storage tissues.

The most significant group of bacteria which take advantage of the vascular channels in the green plant to move rapidly through their hosts are the wilt organisms. A number of bacteria can cause serious vascular wilt diseases, in which the symptoms parallel those caused by fungal pathogens (see Fig. 7.13). These bacteria enter their hosts in diverse ways, such as through wounds created by vectors or cultivation practices, through damaged tissues caused by the emergence of lateral roots or via hydathodes and stomata. Their unicellular morphology then makes them ideally suited for transport within xylem vessels. In some instances, the bacteria then spread rapidly into adjoining parenchyma tissue. In this respect several of these bacterial pathogens differ from the typical fungal vascular wilt pathogens, which do not grow out from the xylem until after the host has died. Vascular wilt bacteria occur in the genera *Corynebacterium, Erwinia, Pseudomonas* and *Xanthomonas*. They are important in both tropical and warm temperate regions and include *Erwinia tracheiphila*, which is responsible for bacterial wilt of wild and cultivated species of the Cucurbitaceae, and *Pseudomonas solanacearum*, which attacks a number of plants including banana (Moko disease), tobacco, tomato and potato.

Colonization by viruses and mycoplasmas

The spread of viruses within their hosts is unique in that they can only multiply within cells and they are small enough to behave as subcellular

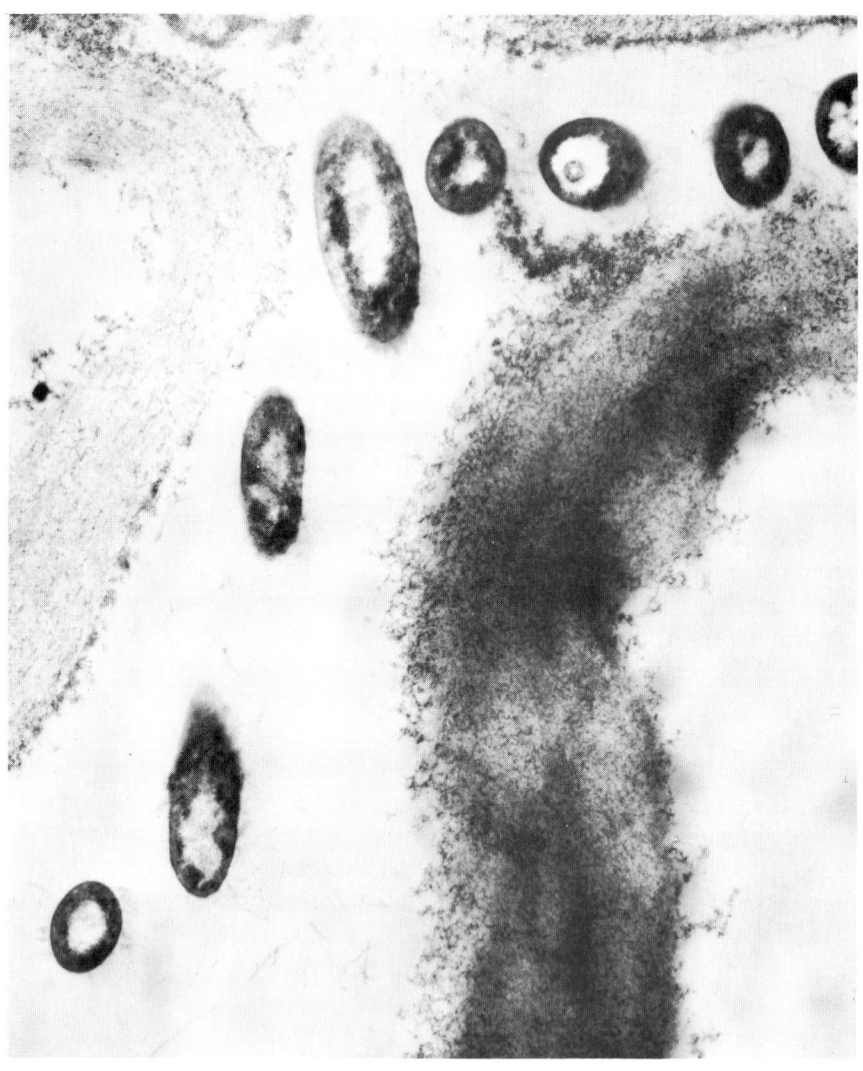

Figure 5.9 Transmission electron micrograph showing *Erwinia* cells in the intercellular spaces of a potato tuber. The tuber cell walls have become swollen due to the macerating activities of the pathogen (× 25 000). (Photograph by R.T. Fox.)

particles. As such they are able to move directly from cell to cell through plasmodesmata; virus particles have been observed within plasmodesmata by electron microscopy. The rate of cell-to-cell spread is fairly low, with the virus taking four or five hours to move from one cell to the next. Much faster spread takes place via the phloem; here the rate of movement has been estimated as high as several centimetres per hour. It is interesting to note that mycoplasmas are almost entirely restricted to phloem elements. Phloem transport (and in a minority of cases xylem transport) plays an important part in the development of virus systemic infections. Literally every cell in the plant may become infected, although the low percentage of infected seed and pollen in most virus diseases suggests that movement into gametophyte tissue or the developing embryo is restricted. Often, meristematic tissues are also virus free; this fact has been put to good use in the production of virus-free plants by meristem culture.

Effect of the environment on colonization

The influence of environmental conditions on the extent to which pathogens spread within the host should also be emphasized. Many pathogens which are normally restricted to a single organ or tissue can, under optimum conditions, become more aggressive and invade further parts of the host. *Botrytis fabae* causes chocolate spot disease of broad beans in which the normal symptom is localized brown lesions on the leaf (see Fig. 2.1). Under some conditions, however, rapidly spreading lesions are formed; the confluence of several such lesions can destroy the whole leaf lamina. Other fungal pathogens may become systemic if they infect the host at a particular stage in its development. For example, *Peronospora parasitica* produces discrete necrotic patches on adult *Brassica* leaves but on seedlings in cold frames it can grow systemically infecting the cotyledons, the hypocotyl and even the root system.

A final word should be added about latent infections where a pathogen is present in a host without causing any visible symptoms. This phenomenon is common with virus diseases and creates problems in the eradication of reservoirs of infection. It is also becoming apparent that many plant tissues contain endogenous bacteria which cause no apparent harm to the host. The relationship of these bacteria to mycoplasma-like organisms is not entirely clear. In some diseases they may contribute to symptoms by becoming active as secondary pathogens.

FURTHER READING

General texts

BLAKEMAN J.P. ed. (1981) *Microbial Ecology of the Phylloplane*. Academic Press, London.
    Useful summaries of the infection procedures adopted by several major groups of pathogens.
MARTIN J.T. & JUNIPER B.E. (1970) *The Cuticles of Plants*. Edward Arnold, London.
    A comprehensive treatment of the external defences which protect the aerial parts of green plants.

Reviews and original papers

COHEN Y. & EYAL H. (1980) Effects of light during infection on the incidence of downy mildew (*Pseudoperonospora cubensis*) on cucumbers. *Physiological Plant Pathology* **17**, 53–62.
MAITI I.B. & KOLATTUKUDY P.E. (1979) Prevention of fungal infection of plants by specific inhibition of cutinase. *Science* **205**, 507–8.
MACNAMARA O. & DICKINSON C.H. (1981) Microbial degradation of plant cuticle. In *Microbial Ecology of the Phylloplane* (ed. Blakeman J.P.), pp. 455–473. Academic Press, London.

WILLIAMS P.H., AIST J.R. & BHATTACHARYA P.K. (1973) Host–parasite relations in cabbage clubroot. In *Fungal Pathogenicity and the Host's Response* (eds Byrde R.J.W. & Cutting C.V.), pp. 144–155, Academic Press, London.

WYNN W.K. & STAPLES R.C. (1981) Tropisms of fungi in host recognition. In *Plant Disease Control* (eds Staples R.C. & Toenniessen G.H.), pp. 45–69. John Wiley & Sons, New York.

6

Host-pathogen interaction at the population level

"Ours is a military campaign against agents that destroy our plants. We cannot wage this campaign successfully without knowing the measure of the enemy's ability to destroy."
K. STARR CHESTER (1906–)

In crop husbandry the fate of the individual plant is often irrelevant. The farmer or forester deals in terms of millions of individuals and only when sufficient numbers succumb to disease is action considered necessary. In the field, therefore, disease is a phenomenon to be considered in terms of populations.

We have already seen how difficult it is to define accurately and describe disease in individual hosts. A similar problem exists in trying to assess the amount of disease in a population of crop plants. Analysis of a disease outbreak demands, however, that there is a satisfactory means whereby the level of disease can be estimated. Such an analysis is necessary if the effects of a disease outbreak on the eventual yield or quality of a crop are to be understood.

Monitoring the occurrence of a particular disease in an individual crop over several years can provide clues as to factors regulating its incidence and severity. This information can then be used to devise predictive systems which forecast the incidence of future outbreaks of the disease. The development of such forecasting systems is especially important for diseases of economically important crop plants which regularly increase to epidemic proportions.

DISEASE ASSESSMENT

The identification of disease in a particular crop may in itself be of little interest to the grower. The subsequent progress of the disease, the possible losses which it may eventually inflict, and the likelihood of it spreading to adjacent fields, are issues of far greater concern than the mere presence of a specific pathogen. These issues also transcend the interests of individual farmers and they demand the collection and collation of data on a country-wide basis. Such disease monitoring may be concerned with a specific disease or the complex of diseases which affect a particular crop. A wide range of methods are used to gain information, including systematic surveys (usually by Government pathologists), aerial photography, planting trap nurseries and encouraging farmers to inspect their crops at regular intervals. For a number of diseases these data are now collated by computer and regular reports, especially via the media, further enhance the general level of awareness about impending epidemics.

The potential severity of a disease outbreak is dependent upon the outcome of infection in individual plants and the capacity of the pathogen to spread through the crop. One is thus faced with a complex situation involving a number of factors: the resistance of the host; the virulence of the pathogen; and the effects of the environment on both these qualities as well as its effects upon the reproduction and dispersal of the pathogen. Superimposed on these interactions there is the additional consideration of the stage in the life cycle of the crop plant at which infection occurs. For instance, a wheat plant is likely to be killed outright by the take-all pathogen if infection occurs prior to tillering (Fig. 6.1), whereas later infections merely result

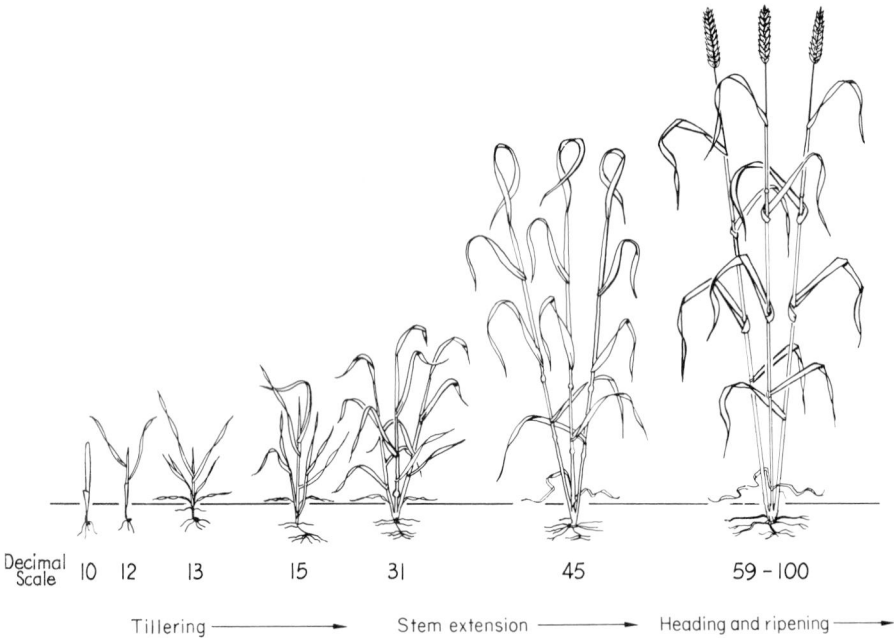

| Decimal Scale | 10 | 12 | 13 | 15 | 31 | 45 | 59 – 100 |

Tillering ⟶   Stem extension ⟶   Heading and ripening ⟶

Figure 6.1   Growth stages in cereals (after Large, 1954). The decimal scale, which ranges from 0 to 100, is used to describe the growth stage of the crop in a semi-quantitative manner.

in a drastic reduction in the size of the grains which are formed. Similarly maize smut kills seedlings but infections of the mature plant only result in unsightly galls which either have a local effect on the host's physiology or destroy individual grains (Fig. 6.2).

Any component of the environment may influence the progress of a disease outbreak. Climatic conditions are of particular importance but they are, of course, notoriously difficult to predict with any accuracy. Soil nutri-

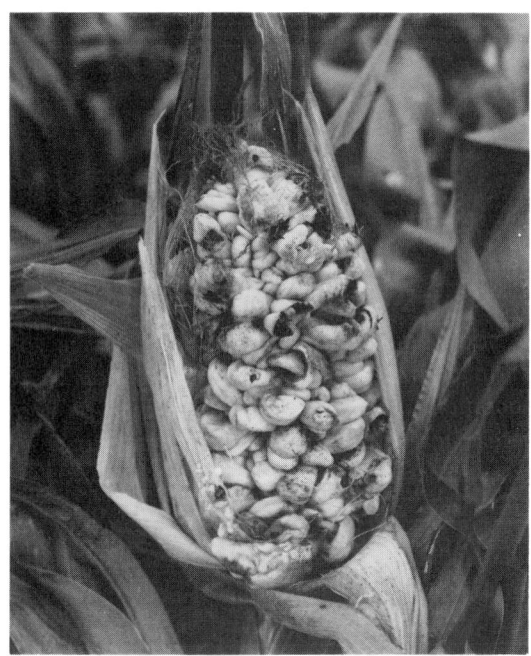

Figure 6.2 Gall symptoms caused by the corn smut pathogen, *Ustilago maydis*, on a maize cob (photograph by courtesy of I.C.I., Plant Protection Division).

ents may influence disease expression in a variety of ways; nitrogen deficiency may impair the host's ability to make good tissue damage due to disease (e.g. the capacity to produce adventitious roots or new leaves may be reduced, while high nitrate levels can result in the development of hosts with low resistance to disease). Such a change has been demonstrated in powdery mildew disease of barley. Increasing amounts of nitrogen fertilizer result in an increased number of infections as related to the number of appressoria, larger colonies and a greater spore production per colony. Thus a cultivar which initially exhibits a high level of resistance may be transformed into one which is highly susceptible. The significance of the nonpathogenic microbes which live on and in the vicinity of host plants is only just beginning to be appreciated. The saprophytic microflora present around plant roots may affect the growth of epiphytic pathogens and it may even determine the relative success of root pathogens such as *Gaeumannomyces* and *Heterobasidion*.

Climatic, edaphic and biotic factors play a major part in determining the rate of reproduction of pathogens and extent of their dispersal to new host plants. In this respect another important factor is the availability of suitable hosts. Systems of monoculture on a plantation, field or glasshouse scale generally ensure an ample supply or concentration of potential hosts. In addition, it is likely that the same crop will be grown widely in the immediate geographic region. This is in part a reflection of the suitability of the soil and climate for particular plants, but the growers choice of crop will also be influenced by the availability of labour, processing plants and government subsidy schemes. Similar pressures have also led to increased genetic uniformity within a crop, with large-scale planting of only one or a few closely related cultivars each season.

In view of these interlocking factors, predictions of the overall loss which may result from a disease outbreak are likely to be as much a matter of intuition as of rational interpretation of the available facts. Yet such predictions are needed, and may indeed be vital, if appropriate and economically sound control measures are to be instituted. Seed inspection and certification, soil sterilization, selective pruning or roguing, premature harvesting and spray programmes all cost money and this expense must be set against the value of the crop. Hence there is a need for methods which enable disease outbreaks to be located rapidly, their severity measured and their further development predicted.

Disease assessment methods

Outbreaks of disease in relatively large perennial plants, e.g. blackcurrant bushes, apple trees and banana plants, may be monitored by regular visual inspection. With annual crops, such as cereals or potatoes, serious disease or even the death of individual plants is more likely to pass unnoticed. This may be particularly serious, in that a disease outbreak in short-lived plants requires prompt action to prevent it becoming a severe problem. Longer-lived plants may be subject to serious symptoms during one season, but with non-lethal pathogens, natural or artificial checks will often restrict the pathogen and allow a return to near-normal crop yields in succeeding years.

In intensive agricultural systems there is, therefore, a need for regular crop inspection and systematic disease surveys. These may be carried out by the grower, by government officials or by representatives of agrochemical companies. The crop is examined at different growth stages (for example see Fig. 6.1) and samples are taken over the whole area where the crop is grown. Data obtained in this way are collated and the patterns of incidence of disease may then be monitored on a local, national or international basis.

Most methods used for recording the severity of disease outbreaks are based on estimates of disease symptoms or yield losses. For many diseases, intensive study has led to a better understanding of the meaning of individual symptoms and their potential significance at different stages in the host's life cycle (Fig. 6.1).

One of the most intensively studied diseases in this respect is late blight of potato. Initially a key was created which allowed visual assessment to be made of the severity of disease outbreaks (Table 6.1). Following a long series of experiments which enabled the vagaries of the weather in any one year to be compensated for, these assessments were related to actual yield losses by comparing diseased plants with others kept healthy by fungicide treatment. The tuber weight losses resulting from severe blight epidemics clearly depend upon the time in the season when infection occurs (Fig. 6.3). This is predictable inasmuch as bulking of tubers is a long-term process and destruction of foliage late in the season will have little appreciable effect on

Table 6.1 Key for the assessment of potato late blight (from the *Transactions of the British Mycological Society*, 1947).

Description of crop	Percentage of crop diseased
Not seen on field	0
Only a few plants affected here and there; up to one or two spots in 12 m radius	0.1
Up to ten spots per plant, or general light spotting	1
About fifty spots per plant or up to one leaflet in ten attacked	5
Nearly every leaflet with lesions, plants still retaining normal form; field may smell of blight, but looks green although every plant affected	25
Every plant affected and about one-half of leaf area destroyed by blight; field looks green flecked with brown	50
About three-quarters of leaf area destroyed by blight; field looks neither predominantly brown nor green. In some varieties the youngest leaves escape infection so that green is more conspicuous than in varieties like King Edward, which commonly shows severe shoot infection	75
Only a few leaves left green, but stems green	95
All leaves dead, stems dead or dying	100

yield. As an aside, an interesting comparison can be made with wheat, where grain filling is a short-term and late event in the development of the crop; direct and drastic effects on yield can be related to disease outbreaks affecting those photosynthetic tissues which are still active just prior to harvest.

Disease assessment keys have been constructed for many pathogens and their use for particular diseases has been standardized to ensure that assess-

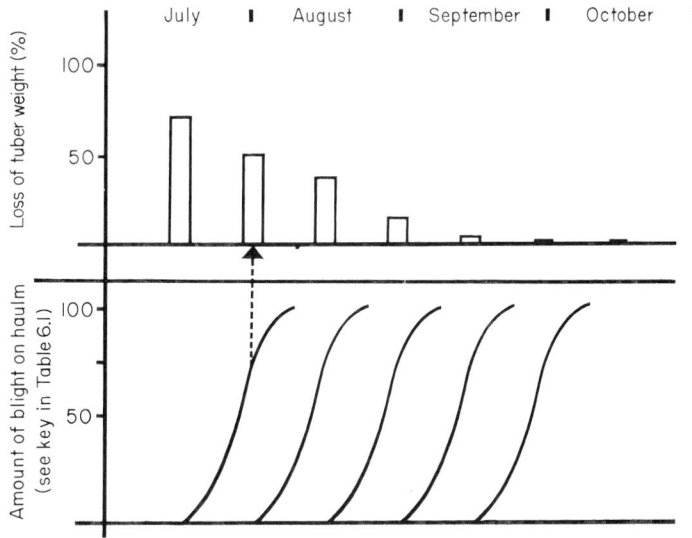

Figure 6.3 Relation between late blight progress and yield loss of potato cultivar Majestic (data from Large, 1952).

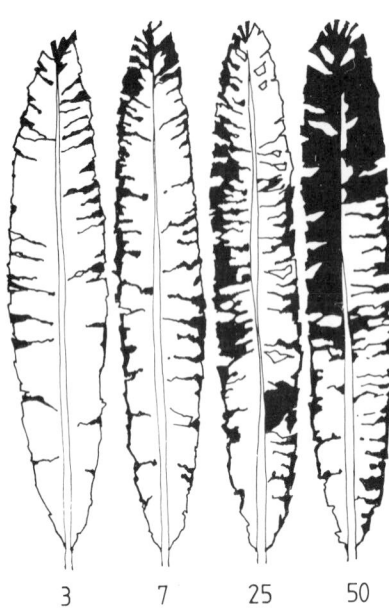

Banana leaf spot

Used for: Leaf spot (*Mycosphaerella musicola*) of banana (also known as Siga-toka or black leaf-streak disease)

Procedure: Select 100 non-flowering plants and number the leaves on each consecutively from the youngest unfurled leaf (No. 1) Record the presence or absence of spots on each leaf. A disease intensity score can also be recorded for each leaf using the key on the left.

| 3 | 7 | 25 | 50 |

PERCENTAGE SPOTTED TISSUE

Disease intensity/loss relationship: the table below indicates the correlation between disease level and fruit loss.

Average No. of youngest spotted leaf	% plants with spotted leaves younger than leaf No. 8	% spotted plants	Fruit loss	
			Field	Transit
10–12	10	40	None	None
8–9	40–60	100	Up to 10% culled as ripe	Up to 20% ripens or colours in 7 days
5–7	60–80	100	Up to 75% culled for soft fingers or yellow pulp	Over 50% of fruit ripens or turns colour in 7 days

Figure 6.4   Disease assessment key for banana leafspot disease (from Stover, 1973).

ments may be compared. Figures 6.4 and 6.5 show the diagrams currently used to assess the severity of Sigatoka disease and powdery mildew on bananas and cereals respectively.

Disease losses may be purely quantitative, as when cereal mildew or rusts debilitate their hosts, or there may be additional, and indeed over-riding, qualitative effects. Apple scab is now scarcely tolerated by the consumer, and potato common scab and banana sooty mould can, if severe,

84

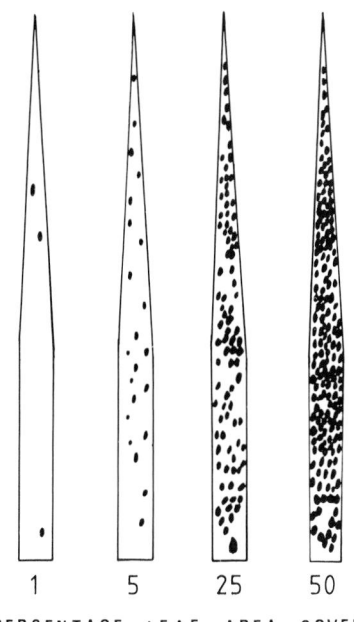

PERCENTAGE LEAF AREA COVERED

Powdery mildew of cereals

Used for: Powdery mildew
(*Erysiphe graminis*) of
barley, oats and wheat.

Procedure: Select a random
sample of fertile tillers,
record disease separately on
each leaf, numbering these
from the top, flag leaf down
the flowering axis.

Growth stages: The key can
be used for recording the
disease at several growth
stages, which should be
carefully noted so that valid
comparisons can be made
between crops and in the
same crop at different dates.

Assessing severity: The area
of the lamina affected by
disease symptoms is recorded on a percentage scale.

Figure 6.5   Disease assessment key for powdery mildew of cereals (from Large & Doling, 1962).

significantly reduce the value of the crop. A further consideration is the effect of some pathogens on the storage properties of the produce. One serious consequence of Sigatoka disease of banana is premature ripening of the fruit in transit, which has obvious economic implications for a tropical crop whose main market is in temperate countries. Even more subtle effects assume significance in products in which quality is of supreme importance. Wine made from grapes affected by grapevine leafroll virus is of inferior quality and colour due to the low sugar and high tartaric acid levels present in diseased grapes at harvest. Disease assessments may thus incorporate analyses of quality as well as the more obvious quantitative estimates. Such qualitative considerations are now assuming greater significance as grading schemes are introduced to benefit both the consumer and the more efficient grower.

As yet physiological and biochemical criteria have not been utilized in this area of pathology. This is not to say that modern technology has failed to provide new techniques for detecting and measuring diseases. Large areas of crops can be surveyed by means of aerial photography and, by using various types of film, diseased plants can be recognized as distinct patches in an otherwise uniform picture (Fig. 6.6). The technique has proved useful with diseases such as late blight of potato, where early DISEASE FOCI can be located and their subsequent spread followed. It is also useful when sudden disaster strikes and a rapid appraisal of the situation is required. Such problems are often made worse by the very large areas involved or by the inac-

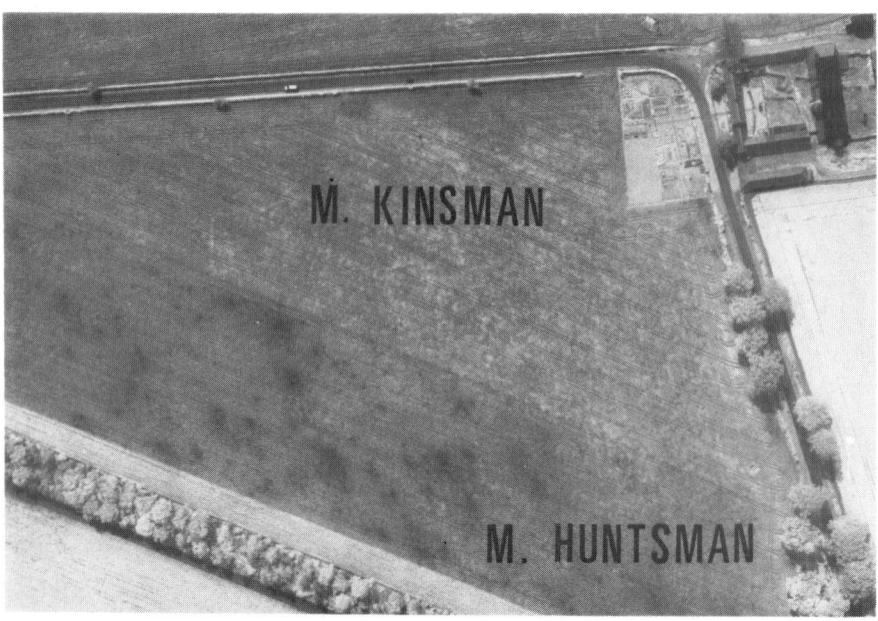

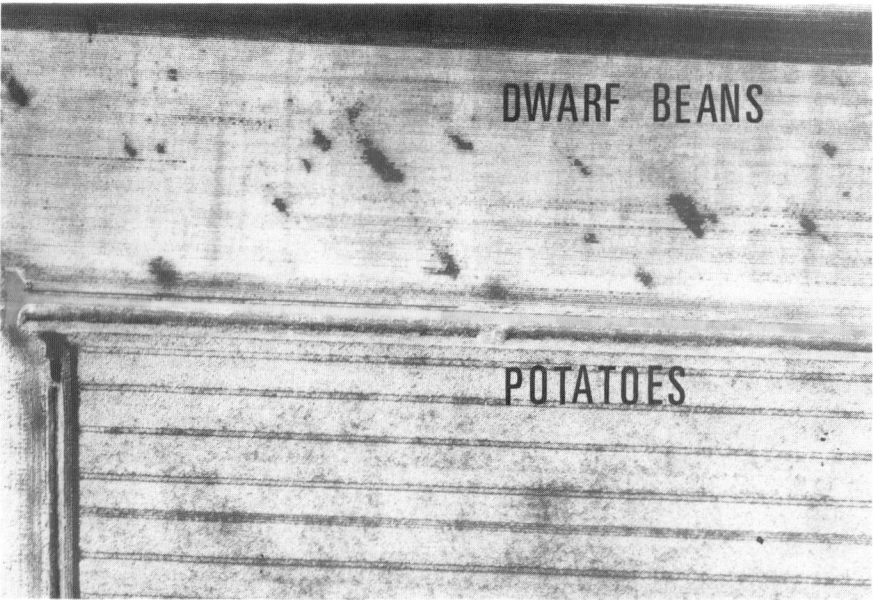

Figure 6.6 Aerial photographs taken with near-infra-red film showing disease patterns in several crops. In the upper photograph an outbreak of yellow stripe rust (*Puccinia striiformis*) is seen in a field containing two cultivars of winter wheat. The disease foci are exclusively confined to the susceptible cultivar, Maris Huntsman, whilst the adjoining Maris Kinsman is unaffected. The foci are elongated in a typical 'fall out' pattern, the direction of which is determined by the prevailing wind. In the lower photograph the dwarf beans are affected by *Pseudomonas phaseolicola* causing halo blight. This pathogen is very effectively spread by rain splash, but only over a limited distance. Hence there are distinct patches in which all the plants are severely affected. In the potato crop, numerous late blight foci can be seen associated with the tractor wheelings. (Photograph Crown Copyright.)

cessibility of the terrain on which the crop is planted. In many parts of the world the wheat crop occupies enormous tracts of land and aerial photography can be used to determine the extent of take-all damage. Similarly, the incidence of *Heterobasidion* can be monitored in pine plantations covering undulating, rocky or boggy land.

DISEASE FORECASTING

Because disease assessment includes a predictive element it is closely linked with disease forecasting. The latter, however, predicts whether or not disease will actually occur as well as estimating the likely extent of its progress through a crop. As outbreaks of certain diseases show a marked correlation with particular climatic conditions, forecasting is often thought of as being synonymous with analysis of the effects of weather on disease epidemics. Many of the more elaborate forecasting systems are based on meteorological data, but it is important to realize that other factors are involved. In its simplest form, forecasting merely relies on knowledge of whether a disease has occurred before in the area concerned. For instance, many farmers know through experience that crops grown in certain fields will be particularly prone to disease. In the light of this knowledge they avoid planting susceptible crops in those fields. Similarly, information on the relative resistance of different cultivars to the prevalent races of a pathogen can be used to ensure that disease is avoided. Agricultural advisory agencies or extension services carry out screening programmes to determine the distribution of races of destructive pathogens such as the cereal rusts and mildews. Patterns of occurrence of disease in the recent past can provide an indication as to the amount of infective material, or inoculum, in the environment. The presence of other host plants, such as the alternate hosts of rust fungi or alternative hosts for viruses, may also be a determining factor.

Diseases which are introduced in seed or other propagules may be forecast by measuring the extent of any contamination in laboratory or greenhouse tests carried out prior to planting the crop. In many countries, seed testing is routinely conducted to provide certification guaranteeing the product's fitness for use. A major problem, with such schemes is that it is often difficult to relate levels of seed contamination to the subsequent development of epidemics, and hence to determine acceptable maximum limits above which seed must either be treated or be rejected. Some such relationships have been established, for example with halo blight of *Phaseolus* beans which are tested for the presence of this bacterium by utilizing its fluorescence characteristics and by serological tests. Field studies have shown that seed samples of *Phaseolus* should have less than 0.025% infection if serious epidemics are to be avoided. This level of seed contamination will give rise to about 0.0025% primary infections, and if the subsequent apparent infection rate (r; see page 97) is 0.15 per infected plant per day, this will lead to about four per cent infection in the mature crop, which is the maximum which can be tolerated before significant losses are experienced.

Other information which may have a bearing on disease forecasts include soil type and local environmental factors, for example, changes in microclimate created by an undulating terrain or the proximity of woods or hedgerows. The intuitive approach of many farmers to avoidance of disease problems will, of course, embrace considerations such as these. After all, man has been growing crops with reasonable success for centuries, for the most part without the advice of plant pathologists!

Climate and disease

Having made all these qualifications, it is still true that for many diseases the dominant factors regulating disease development are those involving the weather. It is possible, in some instances, to establish direct links between climatic conditions and specific processes in the life of the pathogen, for example spore germination or dispersal to new hosts. Furthermore, with some diseases these effects of climate can be narrowed down to one or a few specific components, such as temperature, relative humidity and rainfall. Where the progress of an epidemic can be attributed directly to specific combinations of climatic conditions, monitoring the weather may be sufficient to provide accurate forecasts.

Pseudoperonospora humuli causes downy mildew disease of hops and, in common with other downy mildews, it reproduces asexually by forming sporangia on elongate sporangiophores which protrude through the host's stomata. The formation of these propagules is influenced by relative humidity, which must be >90% for sporulation to occur. Spore release and dispersal are also affected by humidity; the former process requires fluctuating conditions and the latter is only successful if the spores are not subject to desiccation. The final step in the cycle, infection of new hosts, is similarly dependent on favourable environmental factors. Hop leaves must be wet before sporangia can produce zoospores; these swim to stomata, encyst, germinate and penetrate through the aperture (Fig. 5.6).

Correlations between environmental factors and the incidence of hop downy mildew disease outbreaks are not, however, straightforward. Multiple regression analysis has had to be employed to establish an equation which relates the incidence of disease to the amount of rainfall, the duration of leaf-surface wetness (due to rain, but not dew), and airborne-sporangium concentrations (measured by trapping and counting sporangia in known volumes of air). Levels of infection predicted from the equation were compared with actual levels recorded on healthy trap plants exposed in an infected hop garden. A very close agreement was obtained in this test (Fig. 6.7), indicating the potential of such an analytical approach as the basis for short-term forecasting of outbreaks of hop downy mildew.

In discussing the influence of climate on disease expression, it is natural that the emphasis has been put on the significance of regional weather

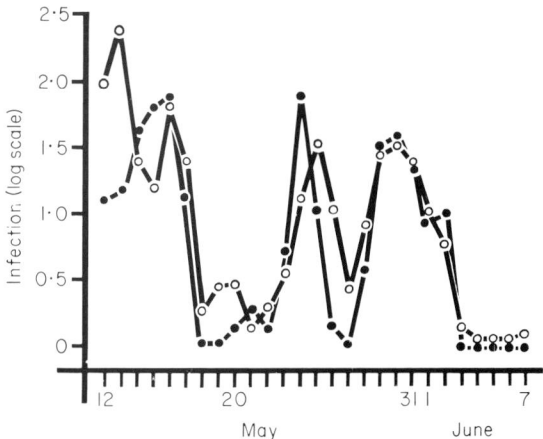

Figure 6.7 Predicted (○) and actual (●) values for infection of hop plants by *Pseudo-peronospora humuli*. Batches of healthy plants were exposed in a disease-affected hop garden at daily intervals and infection subsequently assessed. (Data from Royle, 1973.)

patterns, as described by standard meteorological techniques. In many agricultural regimes, however, crop ECOCLIMATES afford especially favourable conditions for disease development. For example, the environment within the canopy of a mature potato crop is normally far more suitable for the development of blight than the regional weather records would suggest. In particular, the relative humidity in the crop ecoclimate remains very high, long after the air above the canopy has become relatively dry. High humidity is an important requirement for the sporulation of *Phytophthora infestans* and also increases the chances of successful reinfection of new host plants. The discovery of the existence of this extremely favourable environment led to the observation that, in this respect, the crop almost seems to be bent on its own self destruction!

Meteorological forecasting systems

Although the relationship between environmental factors and disease may be difficult to unravel, this has not prevented the development of accurate and effective forecasting schemes. Certain diseases are more obvious candidates for forecasting systems than others and characteristics which facilitate the development of such schemes are listed in Table 6.2.

Table 6.2 Factors which are important in the development of meteorological forecasting systems.

(A) The incidence of disease varies with time due, at least in part, to differences in weather factors.
(B) Experimental studies have shown which weather factors affect the pathogen and the disease.
(C) The disease is economically important.
(D) Economically viable preventative or curative control measures are available.

In England, potato blight warnings were initially based on the recognition of a 'Beaumont period', defined as a period of 48 hours duration over which the temperature remains above 10°C and the relative humidity does not fall below 75%. More recently, a simplified system has been employed in which blight warnings are broadcast if the minimum temperature remains at or above 10°C for 48 hours, during which period the humidity is at 90% or more for at least 11 hours. These 'Smith periods' allow outbreaks of late blight to be forecast in maincrop potatoes in the UK with an acceptable degree of accuracy using macroclimatic, meteorological-station data. The combination of temperature and humidity specified allows the fungus to reproduce, spread and re-infect adjacent plants and hence continue the build-up towards an epidemic. It is obvious, however, that the significance of a Smith period will vary depending on the stage in the life cycle of the potato plant at which it occurs and the extent to which the pathogen is already established. Such considerations have led to the recognition of 'zero dates', before which time disease outbreaks are either rare or of little significance in the build-up of epidemics. Hence, in practical agricultural terms, spells of weather conducive to disease development occurring before a zero date are usually disregarded. However, it has become clear that the early progress of a pathogen may be significant later on, and it is therefore advisable that disease progress is charted throughout the entire season. Information from such a study may determine the extent of the action required when the weather favours the disease at a later, more critical, stage in the crop's development.

More sophisticated, computerized systems for providing short-term warnings of late-blight attacks have been developed in both the USA and West Germany. The American system, which is known as Blitecast, emphasizes the participation of individual farmers. Growers are encouraged to maintain thermohydrographs in their potato fields and when a forecast is required, information from these instruments is telephoned to a central office. It is then fed into a computer programmed with data akin to the Beaumont or Smith criteria and an immediate response is obtained. This includes both a blight warning and a spray recommendation. In the German scheme, Phytprog, emphasis is placed on the provision of negative forecasts, which mean that no action need be taken to control the disease for a specified period—such negative forecasts can usefully limit the costs of control measures as well as keeping environmental damage to a minimum.

All these forecasting systems involve more or less simple models based on actual weather observations. The progress of apple scab, downy mildew of grapevine and a number of other diseases has also been related to similar, relatively simple observations. However, in all these models, the weather favouring a disease outbreak has already arrived when forecasts are made and control measures must be applied relatively quickly following a disease warning. Delay will allow the pathogen to penetrate new hosts and so avoid the toxic effects of conventional protectant pesticides. More sophisticated and commercially useful forecasts are likely to be obtained in the future by using synoptic weather charts, which indicate the likely sequence of meteorological events in succeeding days, weeks or even months. Such information is already used in some forecasting systems, such as that used for potato blight in Ireland. Long-term forecasts are much more valuable than short-term systems, as control measures may then be integrated with other agricultural practices. They are thus more likely to be economically viable. Forecasting will also indicate the fate of pesticides which could be applied and in particular whether they are likely to be still present on the crop at harvest. Even longer term weather predictions may indicate possible trends in disease over several future seasons, and these might influence the choice of cultivar or even of the crop itself.

The discovery of fungicides which have a measure of curative activity has to some extent obviated the need for prior warning of pathogen spread. One of the first examples of such action was seen with dodine, which can eradicate incipient apple scab infections if applied within 48 hours of spore germination. A more recent example concerns the systemic acylalanine metalaxyl, which can destroy potato blight infections if applied shortly after the pathogen has become established in its host tissues (but see Chapter 10 regarding this fungicide). It is envisaged that there will be a growing demand for such compounds, as meteorological forecasting does not yet provide a sufficiently accurate basis on which to plan a programme of control measures.

Population studies

Most of the forecasting schemes discussed above relate to comparatively short-term predictions covering one or two seasons. Increasing efforts are, however, being made to examine long-term changes in pathogen populations. In particular, the changing patterns of virulence factors are being monitored in some pathogens, with a view to pre-empting potentially disastrous epidemics (see Chapter 10). For instance, in the UK the yellow stripe rust population (*Puccinia striiformis*) is analysed annually by growing sets of differential cultivars in trap nurseries at a number of widely spaced sites in the wheat-growing parts of the country. Information from analyses carried out in previous seasons permits predictions to be made as to the likely level of disease on each cultivar. Where the amount of disease is significantly greater than expected, a sample of the pathogen is sent to a central laboratory for further testing. Experiments in controlled environments are then carried out to confirm the occurrence of new virulence factors. Greater flexibility is possible within such a scheme by using mobile trap nurseries, comprising trays of seedlings raised under disease-free conditions. These trays are exposed within the crop and subsequently incubated to encourage disease development. This method is being used to study cereal powdery mildew populations. One drawback with mobile nurseries is that problems arise in keeping plants free from disease over a long growing period and in transferring large specimens to the field and back to the laboratory. This

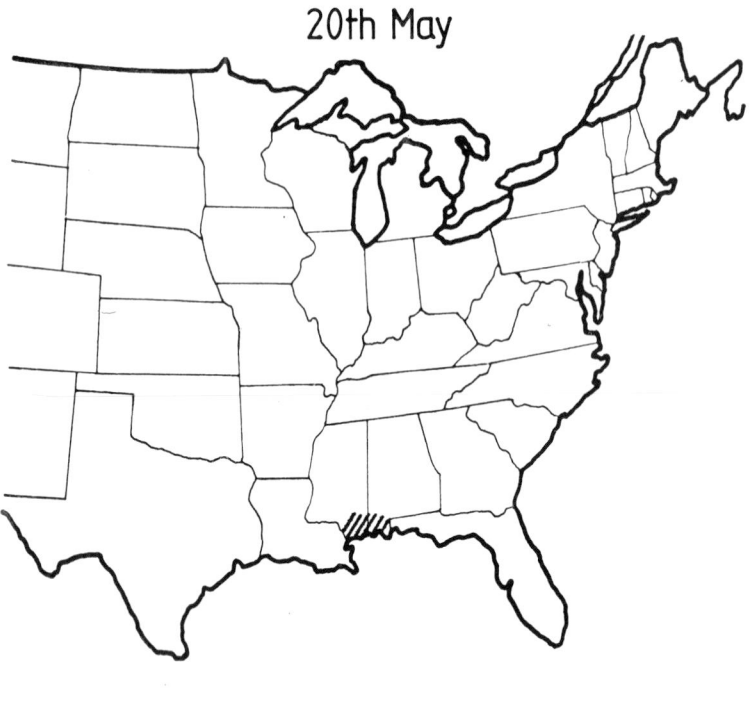

20th May

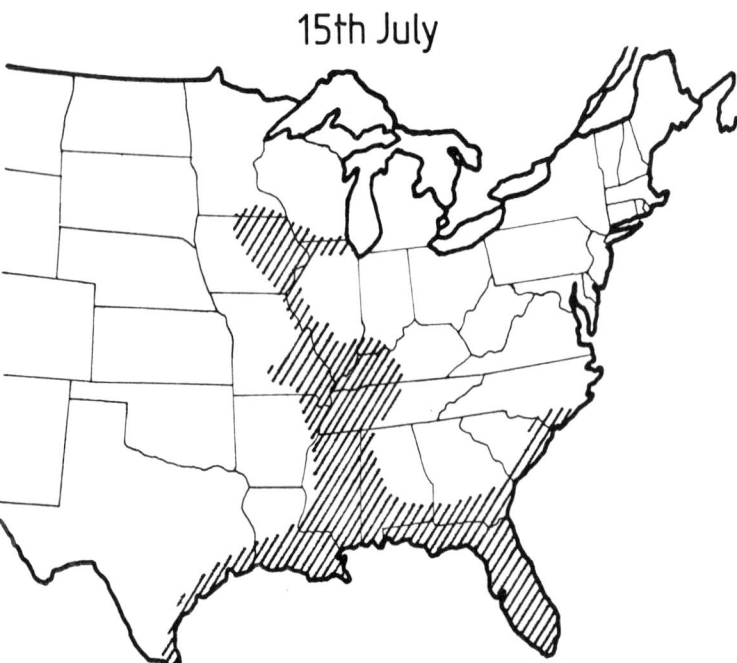

15th July

Figure 6.8 Records of the occurrence of southern corn leaf blight in North America during 1970. The striking progress northwards was assisted by repeated weather patterns involving airstreams from the south. (After Moore, 1970.)

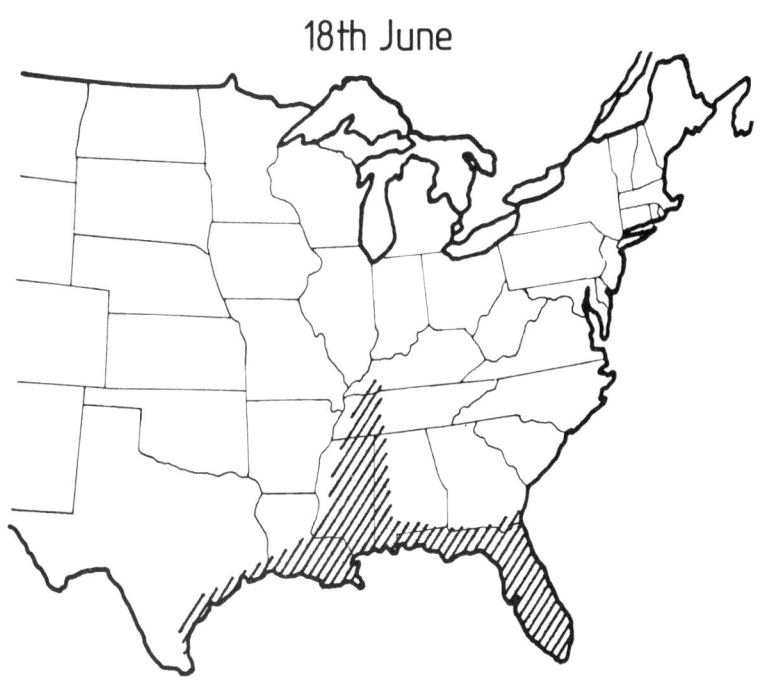

18th June

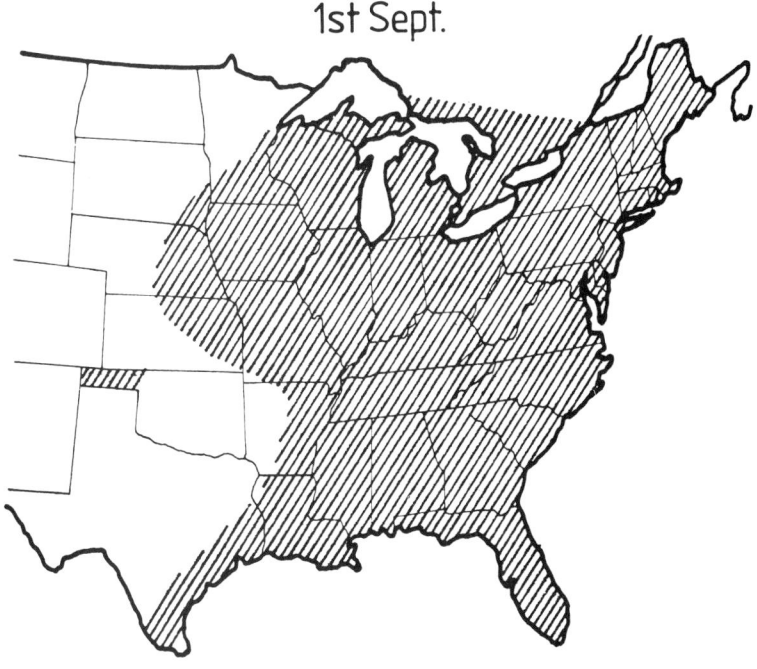

1st Sept.

makes it difficult to search for any effective adult plant resistance, which may be an important component of the crop's ability to withstand disease.

DISEASE EPIDEMICS

Practical recognition of an epidemic implies that there is a progressive increase in the incidence of a particular disease within a defined population of host plants over a time scale which is relevant to the maturation of the crop. Such an epidemic occurring on a continental or global scale is described as a PANDEMIC. There are two components in disease increase: multiplication of the pathogen (i.e. increase in number of individuals) and spread of the pathogen to new hosts. In epidemiology we are therefore concerned with the mechanisms by which the pathogen multiplies and the factors affecting its subsequent dispersal.

In natural plant communities disease epidemics are rare. This is because there are a number of species present in the community and there is considerable genetic variation in natural populations of a single species. Usually, host plants are spatially separated from one another, reducing the opportunities for the pathogen to spread. Individuals within natural host populations also exhibit considerable variations in their ability to resist infection. Where host and pathogen have co-existed for thousands of years it is reasonable to suggest that some form of equilibrium will have evolved between the two organisms. The appearance of new races of the pathogen, through mutation and genetic recombination (see Chapter 4), will sooner or later be countered by the natural selection of host plants which possess corresponding resistance genes.

The domestication or selection of plants for human use has inevitably tended to upset this balance. Cultivation of a single crop species has loaded the odds in favour of the pathogen by providing large stands of similar hosts within which dispersal is likely to be very efficient. Similarly, commercial pressures have lessened the diversity found in natural populations, resulting in the large-scale cultivation of genetically similar individuals. These monocultures provide an ideal situation for the epidemic spread of pathogens, and genetic uniformity is now seen as a major hazard in modern agriculture. A spectacular example of such spread was seen in the infamous epidemic of southern corn leaf blight which in 1970 affected some 85% of the total USA corn acreage. The rapid and extensive movement of this pathogen is charted in Fig. 6.8. Fortunately the situation did not repeat itself in 1971 and an effective level of resistance has subsequently been re-introduced into the crop.

A disease epidemic can only occur if three basic requirements are satisfied.

(1) A large number of host plants are available at a suitable stage of development.

(2) There is a source of virulent inoculum.

(3) Environmental conditions favour growth and spread of the pathogen.

We have already seen that agriculture provides the first requirement for an epidemic to occur. INOCULUM, the portion of a pathogen that is transmitted to or grows into contact with a new host, may be present either as airborne or soil-borne propagules, or may already occur in contaminated seed or other plant propagation material. The actual infection of a host by the pathogen, and the subsequent development of the pathogen to the stage at which new inoculum is produced, is dependent upon environmental conditions.

The two latter components, virulent inoculum and favourable environment, are often embraced in the concept of INOCULUM POTENTIAL. Although there is dispute about the precise meaning of this term, it is essentially a measure of the biological energy available for the colonization of the host. The concept is useful because it draws attention to the fact that disease development is influenced by a multitude of factors. For our purposes it is important to distinguish between the intensity factor, i.e. the number of infective propagules present, which is sometimes termed the INOCULUM DENSITY, and the capacity factor or INFECTION POTENTIAL. The latter is a measure of the ability of individual propagules to cause disease under the prevailing conditions. Environmental factors capable of influencing the progress of an epidemic include temperature, relative humidity, dew formation, rainfall, photoperiod, windspeed and direction, sunshine duration and soil pH. In other words, anything which affects either the development of the pathogen or the performance of the host will influence a disease epidemic.

The disease growth curve

If one plots the amount of disease in a crop against time, one obtains graphs such as those shown in Fig. 6.9. The examples here comprise data from potato late blight epidemics, but similar disease growth curves can be obtained for a variety of plant diseases. All epidemics share this common factor of dynamic increase; the time scale may vary, however, from a few weeks to many years. Potato late blight and the cereal rusts are typical of

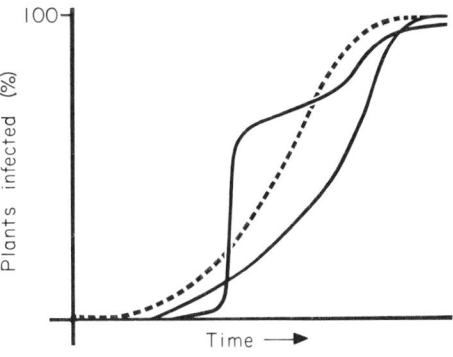

Figure 6.9 An ideal epidemic progress curve (– – –) compared with two actual disease progress curves for potato late blight (data from James *et al.*, 1972).

airborne diseases in which a high rate of pathogen multiplication and dispersal can lead to an explosive epidemic. The idealized disease growth curve is sigmoid (Fig. 6.9), similar to the classic biological growth curve describing the growth of an individual or the multiplication of a bacterial culture. One can distinguish three phases of the curve, an initial lag, a phase of exponential increase and a final decline.

What factors determine this shape? The initial lag phase is primarily due to the small amount of inoculum present at the start of an epidemic. In the case of potato blight, the fungus overwinters in seed tubers or discarded tubers left in piles known as cull heaps. Epidemics are initiated by sporangia formed on diseased shoots developing from such tubers. At first there may be very few affected host plants in the population; a high proportion of these disease foci will be passing through the LATENT PERIOD between infection of the host and production of new infective propagules by the pathogen. Once the amount of inoculum has increased, however, the epidemic moves into the exponential phase. The availability of inoculum is no longer limiting and there are still numerous disease-free hosts within the crop. In this phase the increase in amount of disease is logarithmic. Eventually, the rate of disease increase begins to fall and the epidemic declines. There may be several reasons for this, including the limited number of hosts available for infection and the onset of unfavourable environmental conditions. In the case of potato blight, the pathogen may literally exhaust the supply of host plants.

Mathematical description of epidemics

In Fig. 6.9 we obtained sigmoid epidemic curves by plotting numbers of diseased plants against time. A more exacting interpretation of the central, logarithmic phase of these curves may be obtained by plotting the natural logarithm (ln) of the quantity of disease (q) against time (t) (Fig. 6.10). For this purpose the quantity of disease may be measured in any convenient

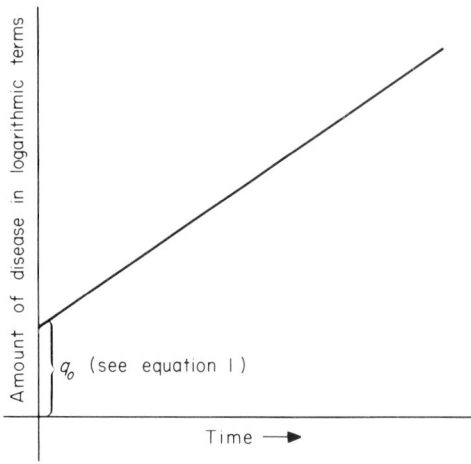

q_0 (see equation 1)

Time →

Amount of disease in logarithmic terms

Figure 6.10
Disease increase
with time plotted on a
logarithmic scale.

way, including number of plants infected, area of leaf or other tissue colonized, or weight loss as compared with control plants. The straight line which is obtained may be characterized by the equation:

$$\ln q = rt + \ln q_0 \tag{1}$$

where r is a constant and q_0 is the quantity of disease present in the crop at the start of the epidemic. By eliminating logarithms this equation becomes:

$$q = q_0 e^{rt} \tag{2}$$

where e is the exponential constant (the base for natural logarithms).

The vital factor in these formulae, in terms of its significance in different host–pathogen–environment combinations, is r. We can obtain a value for r in any field situation by measuring the amounts of disease present (q_1, q_2) at times t_1 and t_2 during the logarithmic phase of disease spread. Equation 1 may then be rewritten:

$$\ln q_1 = rt_1 + \ln q_0 \tag{3}$$

$$\text{and} \quad \ln q_2 = rt_2 + \ln q_0 \tag{4}$$

If equation 3 is subtracted from equation 4 then:

$$\ln q_2 - \ln q_1 = r(t_2 - t_1)$$

$$\text{or} \quad r = (\ln q_2 - \ln q_1)\,\frac{1}{t_2 - t_1} \tag{5}$$

An important qualification must, however, be made in applying these equations. They only hold if there is no restriction of the development of the pathogen. In practice, of course, the population of healthy plants must be declining as q increases. This limitation can be compensated for by taking disease amounts as $q/(1 - q)$, that is, quantity of diseased material over the remaining quantity of healthy material [this becomes $q/(100 - q)$ if disease is expressed in percentage terms]. Equation 5 may then be expressed:

$$r = \left[\ln \left(\frac{q_2}{1 - q_2} \right) - \ln \left(\frac{q_1}{1 - q_1} \right) \right] \frac{1}{t_2 - t_1}$$

$$\text{or} \quad r = \ln \frac{q_2(1 - q_1)}{q_1(1 - q_2)} \times \frac{1}{t_2 - t_1}$$

Epidemic modelling

The implications of these mathematical models of disease development have been extensively explored by van der Plank and others. It is essential that such models are valid and reliable, and that they are orientated towards a clearly defined goal. In addition, they should be simple in construction, logical and mathematically correct. Several types of model are used in epidemiology (Table 6.3). Descriptive models allow for the presentation of experimental data, which may be orientated towards the proof of a hypoth-

Table 6.3 Mathematical models used in epidemiology (after Kranz & Royle, 1978).

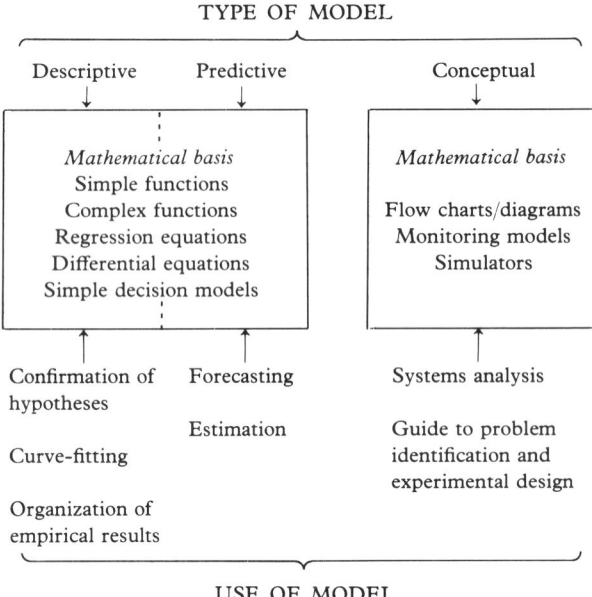

TYPE OF MODEL

		Conceptual
Descriptive	Predictive	

Mathematical basis
Simple functions
Complex functions
Regression equations
Differential equations
Simple decision models

Mathematical basis

Flow charts/diagrams
Monitoring models
Simulators

Confirmation of hypotheses	Forecasting	Systems analysis
	Estimation	Guide to problem
Curve-fitting		identification and experimental design
Organization of empirical results		

USE OF MODEL

esis. Predictive models are a subdivision of the descriptive approach, in which the emphasis is placed on those variables which have the greatest value in foretelling the likely course of events. Conceptual models involve an element of simplification in that all the mechanisms of the epidemic are represented by a single model or a series of linked sub-models.

Examples of descriptive models abound, although they are not necessarily thought of in this context. A simple hypothesis described in mathematical terms is the epidemic threshold theorum. If i = the infectious period, i.e. the time during which a lesion is producing spores, and R_c = the basic infection rate, i.e. the number of new lesions produced per day, then an epidemic will commence when $iR_c > 1$.

Predictive models often involve the use of the apparent infection rate r. Measurements of r can be used to determine the likely advantage of sanitation measures, which reduce the initial inoculum, and fungicide treatments, which reduce the infection rate. Furthermore, the impact of different resistance genes, either exposed alone or in combination, on the progress of an epidemic can be assessed by making measurements of r in various cropping schemes.

Conceptual models attempt to simulate the whole process of epidemic development. For example, EPIMAY provides an account of epidemics of southern corn leaf blight, and EPIDEM is a programme modelling epidemics of early blight of potato. In both these systems the infection cycle of the pathogen is described in qualitative and quantitative terms and the biological and environmental factors affecting each stage in the process are added into the computer programme. If data on weather and crop development are then presented to the computer, it will provide a forecast. Despite the obvious attractions of such systems it must be noted that such simulators are only as good as the quality of the basic data on which they are founded and there is still a distinct shortage of such information for many important pathogens. These simulations have, however, the virtue of exposing deficiencies in our knowledge of the interactions between host and pathogen under field conditions.

Compound- and simple-interest disease

For epidemics where the pathogen passes through several generations in one growing season, and where each generation produces further inoculum, van der Plank has coined the term COMPOUND-INTEREST DISEASE. Because each diseased plant is capable of producing yet more infective material, the epidemic progresses by ever larger increments, in the same way as a compound-interest savings account generates interest upon interest. Examples of this type of epidemic are provided by many of the airborne, foliar pathogens, such as the rusts, mildews and potato blight, where each spore is capable of initiating a lesion in which further sporulation occurs. On susceptible hosts under favourable environmental conditions, the multiplication of the pathogen is very rapid and consequently the rate of disease increase r reaches a high value.

It is possible to contrast compound-interest diseases with others where all the infections occurring in a season are derived from inoculum present at the beginning of the season. This is typically the case with soil-borne pathogens, for instance, the vascular wilt fungi where an increase in the number of diseased plants as the season advances is not primarily due to the reproduction of the pathogen or its growth from one infected plant to other uninfected individuals. Increase in disease with time in this instance is not logarithmic and such epidemics can be described as SIMPLE-INTEREST DISEASE. However in perennial crops or where continuous planting with one crop is practised, the level of simple-interest disease may increase over a number of years with ultimately disastrous effects. This pattern is seen in a variety of plantation crop diseases, notably Panama disease of banana caused by *Fusarium oxysporum* f.sp. *cubense* and in some viral diseases of soft fruits, for example raspberry ringspot. A similar inexorable increase in a simple-interest disease can also occur in an annual crop when the pathogen is dispersed in or on the seed, as is seen with the cereal smuts.

Van der Plank points out that another way of thinking about these two types of epidemic is in terms of the relative birth rates and death rates of the pathogens involved. Pathogens causing simple-interest diseases have characteristically low birth rates, but their propagules often remain viable for long periods. These can, therefore, be considered as low-death-rate diseases, as opposed to compound-interest diseases which are called high-birth-rate diseases. In the latter, the important feature of the pathogen involved is its ability to reproduce rapidly. The propagules of such pathogens may be relatively shortlived.

Although the disease growth curve can provide useful generalizations about the progress of an epidemic, it is inevitably an over-simplification. We have assumed a favourable environment for multiplication and spread of the pathogen. In reality, environmental conditions fluctuate and the progress of an epidemic will be intermittent rather than continuous. Similarly, the spatial distribution of disease will be discontinuous and the rate of increase will differ depending upon the density of uninfected hosts and other factors.

The influence of the environment on the development of an epidemic is complex, with both direct effects on the latent period and indirect effects on the relative resistance of host plants. Temperature has a profound effect on the incubation period between infection and production of further inoculum. For instance, with black stem rust of wheat the disease cycle (from spore to spore) takes 15 days at 10°C, but only 5–6 days at 23°C. Obviously in this case the latent period is reduced at higher temperatures and the epidemic will progress more rapidly. We have already seen that the correlation between relative humidity and disease incidence can be particularly dramatic.

It is also important to appreciate that the progress of an epidemic may be dependent on the date at which it begins. Practical experience shows that if a disease occurs before a certain crop growth stage it will have a far greater impact than later outbreaks. This may simply be because of the time available for the pathogen to multiply and spread during the remainder of the growing season.

RELEVANCE OF EPIDEMIOLOGY TO CONTROL

From our earlier consideration of the three essential ingredients for an epidemic to occur, namely suitable hosts, virulent inoculum and a favourable environment, it should be apparent that rational control measures are aimed at altering one or more of these factors. For instance, one can plant resistant crop varieties, inoculum can be reduced by crop sanitation or seed sterilization, and the environment can be altered in such a way that infection no longer occurs. The use of fungicides or other chemicals may be regarded as examples of ways in which such unfavourable environments can be established. These applied aspects of epidemiology will be discussed further in Chapter 10.

The distinction between simple-interest and compound-interest diseases also has relevance to methods of control. With simple-interest disease the most effective approach is often to reduce the initial inoculum as there is a direct relationship between the inoculum and the amount of disease produced. Fungicidal seed treatments are effective in controlling several cereal smuts because they kill off most of the seed-borne inoculum. However, when dealing with compound-interest diseases merely reducing the initial inoculum is ineffective. This is because in these diseases even a tiny amount of inoculum can quickly multiply to damaging proportions. Control measures for compound-interest diseases are usually designed to prevent the pathogen from generating fresh inoculum. In other words, the latent period between infection and sporulation is increased. This is usually achieved by using fungicides or by growing resistant hosts in which the disease cycle is slowed down. Figure 6.11 shows the effects of various fungicidal sprays on

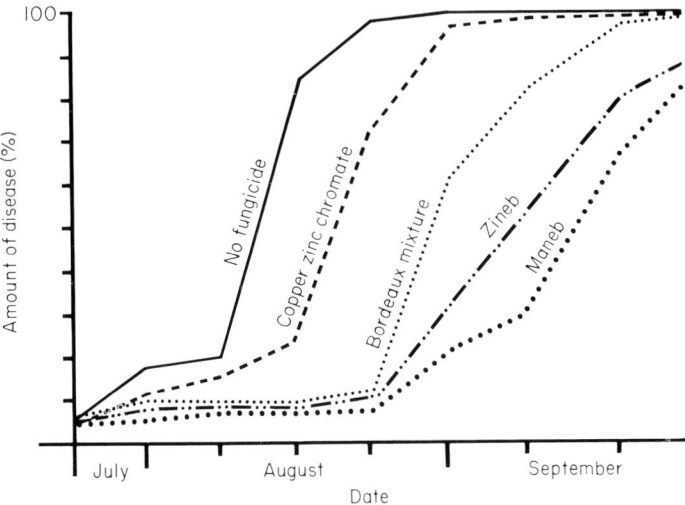

Figure 6.11 Progress of a potato late blight epidemic and the effects of several foliar fungicides applied weekly from mid July (data from Hooker, 1956).

the progress of a potato-blight epidemic. Although none of these actually prevented the epidemic from occurring, the initial lag phase was extended sufficiently to prevent significant reductions in crop yield. When the phase of exponential increase in disease is delayed in this way, bulking-up of the tubers can take place before foliar damage reaches a critical level (Fig. 6.3).

Quarantine

The essential feature of these various strategies is that even though the pathogen is rarely eradicated the progress of an epidemic is delayed. An alternative approach is to try to prevent the pathogen from coming into contact with the crop. In this respect the aim is to avoid pathogens becoming ENDEMIC, that is, permanently established at a moderate or even serious level in a particular geographical area.

A feature of man's domestication of plants has been the introduction of crops into new geographical areas. In some instances these crops have remained free of their most damaging pathogens and it is a matter of concern that this situation should continue. Consequently, strict quarantine meas-

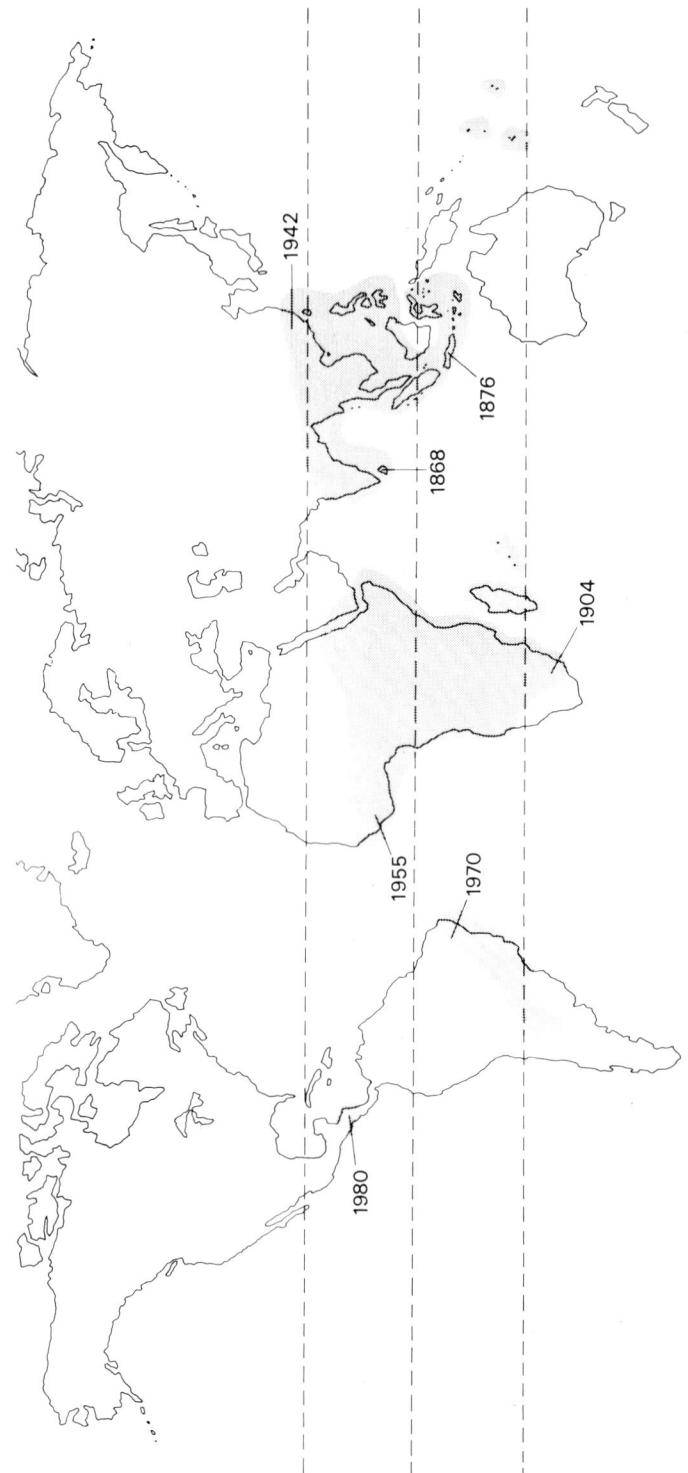

Figure 6.12 Present distribution of the coffee rust fungus, *Hemileia vastatrix*, together with some indications as to its previous movements, as charted by the dates when it was first recorded in various countries (map reproduced by courtesy of the Commonwealth Mycological Institute).

ures are enforced to prevent the introduction of diseases. The cultivation of rubber in Malaysia provides a good example. This tree is a native of the Amazon basin and it was introduced into Malaysia, via the Royal Botanic Gardens at Kew, in the 1870s. Fortuitously, the destructive leaf-blight disease caused by *Dothidella ulei* was not present in the introduced stock and quarantine measures have ensured that the area has remained free from the disease ever since. In South America, leaf blight has effectively prevented the commercial exploitation of the rubber tree.

Similar quarantine schemes operate in most countries, backed up by national and international legislation. The efficacy of such quarantine measures depends, however, on the existence of effective natural barriers, such as oceans and mountain ranges. Even then, exclusion may prove impossible as long-distance dispersal may sometimes occur. It is possible that the appearance of blue mould disease (*Peronospora tabacina*) on European tobacco crops was due to aerial dispersal of spores from America. More recently, the destructive coffee rust disease has dramatically extended its territory to include the major coffee growing regions of South America (Fig. 6.12).

Even in those instances where a disease is endemic to an area it is advantageous to limit the amount of inoculum initially present. One method of doing this is to ensure that all propagation material is free from pathogens. This has long been the aim of testing schemes which assess the extent to which seed is contaminated. The results of these tests can then be used to decide whether the seed or seedlings should be treated with fungicides.

We have already seen that viruses are commonly transmitted by vegetative propagation. For this reason the production of seed potatoes is subject to close scrutiny by government officials. In addition, the possibility of viruses being introduced into the seed stocks themselves is reduced by propagating them in areas which are relatively free from the viruses' normal insect vectors.

In recent years, advances in botanical techniques, such as tissue culture, have been exploited to improve crop hygiene. It is now possible to regenerate unlimited clones of whole plants from excised tissues or even from single cells. Tissue culture techniques have already found practical application in the eradication of viruses from many crops by means of meristem tip culture. An additional advantage of these techniques is the possibility of maintaining virus-free genetic stocks under sterile conditions for an indefinite period. Tissue culture is gradually supplanting the crude traditional methods of vegetative propagation. It is already being used for several ornamentals and for soft fruits such as strawberries.

Disease legislation

For quarantine to be effective it must be backed up by legislation. As an example, potato wart disease (*Synchytrium endobioticum*) (Fig. 7.17ii) has been controlled in the UK by a series of legislative measures which date from 1908. Initially, this pathogen was made a scheduled pest, which meant that farmers had to notify outbreaks to the Ministry of Agriculture. Subsequent government orders prohibited the import of wart-affected potatoes and compelled farmers to grow only resistant cultivars on contaminated land. At present, wart disease occurs only rarely in commercial crops in the UK and outbreaks are mainly confined to plants grown in allotments and gardens.

Continued vigilance is required to prevent other potentially serious diseases from becoming established in new areas. For instance, white rust of chrysanthemums, caused by *Puccinia horiana*, is prevalent in continental Europe but is not currently endemic in the UK. This position is maintained by exclusion measures aimed at preventing the importation of the pathogen. These are enforced by plant health inspectors who visit wholesale flower markets and nurseries dealing in imported cuttings. When outbreaks do occur a stringent eradication policy is adopted.

The unintentional introduction of a new pathogen or a more virulent strain of an endemic pathogen may have serious consequences for the indigenous wild species as well as cultivated crops. The decimation of the European elm population by an introduced strain of *Ceratocystis ulmi* has highlighted this problem and raised fears that similar destructive pathogens, e.g. the oak wilt fungus *Ceratocystis fagacearum*, may follow in its footsteps.

FURTHER READING

General texts

EBBELLS D.L. & KING J.E. eds (1979) *Plant Health*. Blackwell Scientific Publications, Oxford.
An up-to-date appraisal of plant disease legislation, quarantine precautions and eradication schemes.

CHIARAPPA L. ed. (1971) *Crop Loss Assessment Methods*. Published by Food and Agriculture Organisation and Commonwealth Agricultural Bureau.
A collection of keys and assessment methods.

VAN DER PLANK J.E. (1963) *Plant Diseases: Epidemics and Control*. Academic Press, New York.
A pioneering text which laid the basis for most subsequent mathematical analyses of plant disease (e.g. Zadoks & Schein, 1979).

SCOTT P.R. & BAINBRIDGE A. eds (1978) *Plant Disease Epidemiology*. Blackwell Scientific Publications, Oxford.
A useful collection of articles on all aspects of epidemiology.

WHEELER B.E.J. (1976) *Diseases in Crops*. Institute of Biology Studies in Biology No. 64. Edward Arnold, London.
An accessible account of the principles of epidemiology with a strong mathematical ingredient.

ZADOKS J.C. & SCHEIN R.D. (1979) *Epidemiology and Plant Disease Management*. Oxford University Press, Oxford.
Described as a primer in epidemiology and plant-disease management, the emphasis is on fungal pathogens.

Reviews and original articles

BOURKE P.M.A. (1970) Use of weather information in the prediction of plant disease epiphytotics. *Annual Review of Phytopathology* **8**, 345–370.

KRAUSE R.A., MASSIE L.B. & HYRE R.A. (1975) Blitecast: a computerized forecast of potato late blight. *Plant Disease Reporter* **59**, 95–8.

THRESH M.J. (1974) Temporal patterns of virus spread. *Annual Review of Phytopathology* **12**, 111–128.

WAGGONER P.E. (1977) Contributions of mathematical models to epidemiology. *Annals of the New York Academy of Sciences* **287**, 191–206.

WALKEY D.G.A. (1980) Production of virus-free plants by tissue culture. In *Tissue Culture Methods for Plant Pathologists* (eds Ingram D.S. & Helgeson J.P.), pp. 109–117. Blackwell Scientific Publications, Oxford.

YOUNG H.C. JR., PRESCOTT J.M. & SAARI E.E. (1978) Role of disease monitoring in preventing epidemics. *Annual Review of Phytopathology* **16**, 263–285.

7

Host–pathogen interaction at the whole plant and cellular level

"Far from being an insurmountable obstacle to the analysis of an organic system, a pathological disorder is often the key to understanding it"

KONRAD LORENZ (1903–   )

Given favourable environmental conditions, the progress of an epidemic is determined by interactions between individual plants and the pathogen. These interactions at the cellular and molecular level are of fundamental interest, as a better understanding of the processes of disease development may eventually lead to more rational and effective control methods. This has already proved the case with infectious diseases of man, where the discovery of the immune system has facilitated major advances in disease prevention.

Parasitism is a nutritional relationship. The establishment of contact with suitable nutrient substrates in the host is usually a prerequisite for continued development of the pathogen and hence of the disease. The spores of biotrophic fungi, for instance, contain food resources sufficient only for germination and a certain amount of hyphal growth; unless the fungus is able to penetrate living host tissue during this brief phase of independence it will die. This dependence reaches an extreme in the case of viruses. Multiplication and colonization of host tissues can only occur if the virus gains access to the metabolic machinery of the host cell. By contrast, some necrotrophs are able to flourish for an extended period without penetrating their hosts.

The first phase of host–pathogen interaction takes place at or on the surface of the host plant (see Chapter 5). It is worth recalling that some interactions occur before physical contact between the two partners is established; for example, substances diffusing from the host may influence the behaviour of the pathogen. It is unlikely, however, that such stimulatory or inhibitory effects are the sole factors determining whether or not infection takes place. We should also remind ourselves that, strictly speaking, the infection court is not necessarily at the external surface of the host. A comparatively large number of pathogens bypass the host's external barriers by entering through wounds or natural openings. Pathogens carried by vectors are introduced directly into the internal tissues of the host plant, while some seed-borne pathogens avoid the penetration phase altogether by being transmitted through the embryo. These examples serve to show that the initial confrontation in any host–pathogen interaction is not always between a propagule and an intact leaf or root.

When tobacco mosaic virus (TMV) is inoculated into most varieties of tobacco, the virus multiplies and spreads throughout the plant. If the same virus is inoculated into *Nicotiana tabacum* var. *xanthi* or the related species *N. glutinosa,* infection is restricted to small necrotic areas on the leaf, described as local lesions. Similar localization of invasion is seen with many bacterial and fungal pathogens; for instance the majority of leaf-infecting fungi do not invade the whole of the leaf, being instead limited to discrete lesions. What are the reasons for this? How is it that certain plants are able to resist attack by a particular pathogen? Much of what follows in this and the next two chapters is concerned, directly or indirectly, with the answer to this question.

As well as trying to explain differences in resistance to pathogens we also need to consider how the successful pathogen damages the host to give rise to typical disease symptoms. What essential host processes are being disrupted during the course of disease development? A necessary first step towards understanding pathogenesis is to identify these changes in host physiology.

In this chapter we will concentrate on cytological and physiological aspects of host–pathogen relations and place emphasis on the host as an active partner in the interaction.

THE HOST–PATHOGEN INTERFACE

The site of contact between a pathogen and the host cell or protoplasm is known as the host–pathogen interface. This is the site at which materials are taken up or exchanged. At present we have only a limited idea as to the processes occurring at the host–pathogen interface. Nevertheless, in recent years a considerable amount of ultrastructural detail has been revealed by transmission electron microscopy of various host–micro-organism associations. This information has provided valuable insights into the nature of parasitic disease.

The type of host–pathogen interface formed is directly linked with the mode of growth of the pathogen during colonization of the host. Three broad categories may be distinguished (Table 7.1). These categories are not

Table 7.1   Types of host–pathogen interface.

1. Pathogen grows between host cells	Intercellular	e.g. Necrotrophic bacteria and fungi
2. Pathogen grows partially or entirely within host cells		
a. Intercellular hyphae produce intracellular haustoria	Partially intracellular	e.g. Biotrophic fungi
b. Pathogen contained within host cell	Entirely intracellular	e.g. Plasmodial fungi, viruses, mycoplasmas

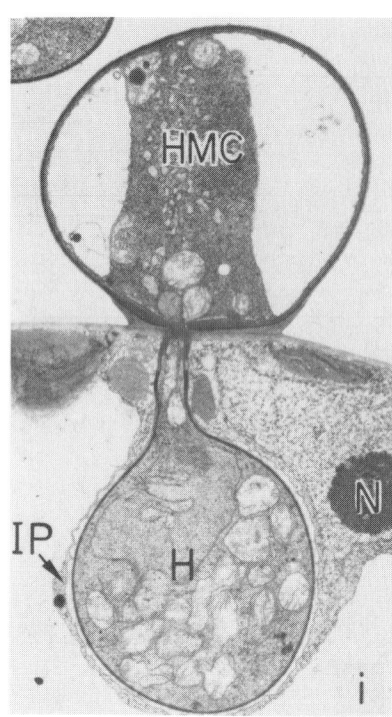

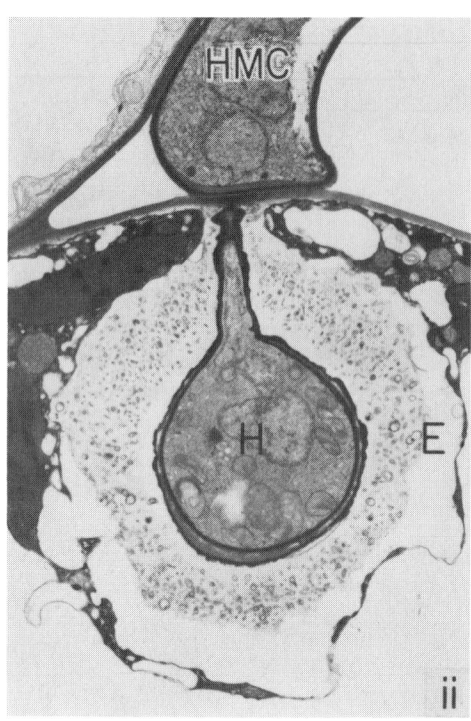

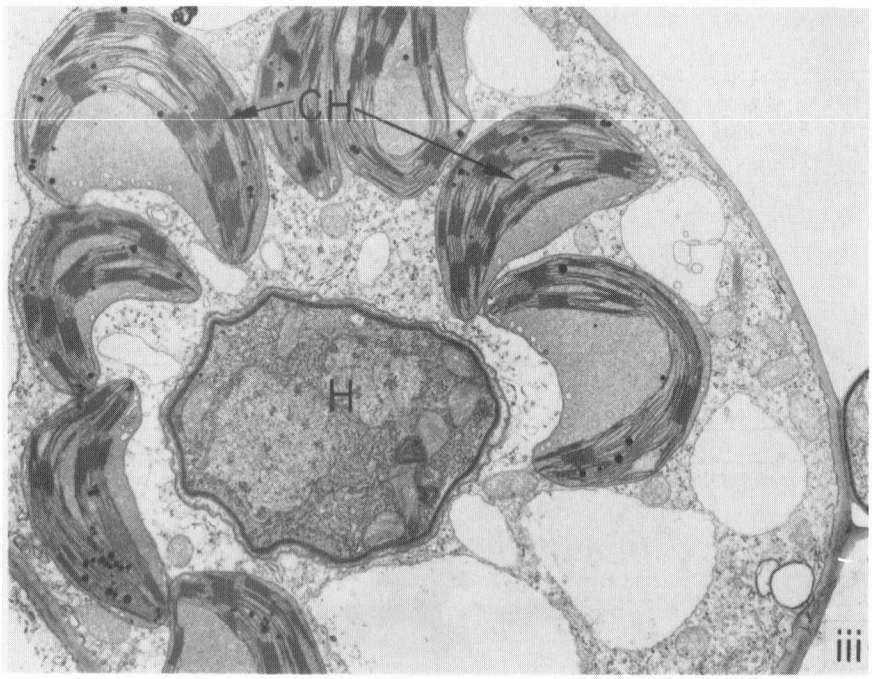

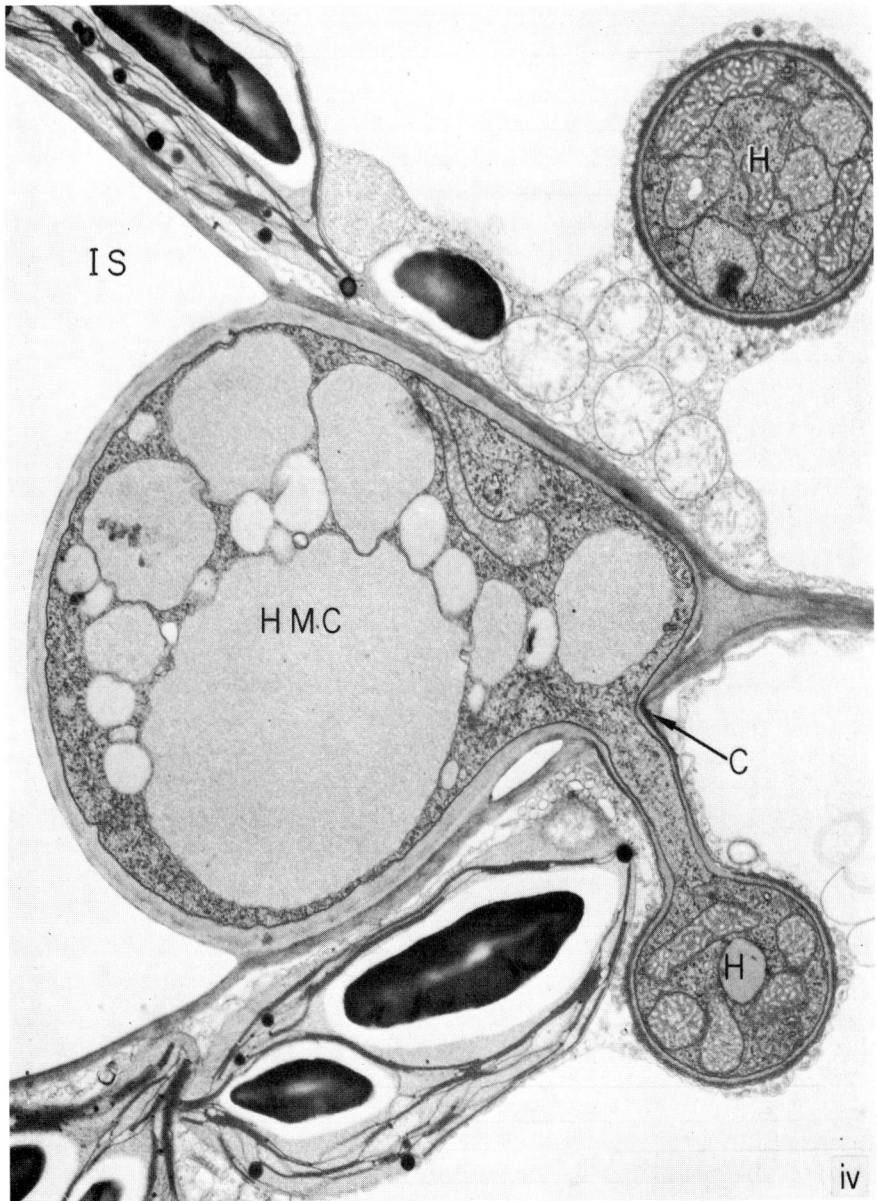

Figure 7.1 Haustoria of fungi in host cells. (**i–iii**) the rust *Melampsora* in flax and (**iv**) white blister rust, *Albugo*, in cabbage. (**i**) 5 day-old compatible reaction (× 7850), (**ii**) 9-day-old resistant reaction showing encapsulation (E) enclosing haustorium, and necrosis of host cytoplasm (× 7850), (**iii**) Haustorium in host mesophyll cell surrounded by chloroplasts (CH) (× 11 000). H = haustorium, HMC = haustorial mother cell, N = host cell nucleus, IP = invaginated plasma membrane, (**iv**) spherical haustorium (H) in host cell, showing haustorial mother cell (HMC) in intercellular space (IS) and collar (C) at penetration site. A second haustorium can be seen in the adjacent host cell (× 16 000). (From Coffey 1975, 1976.)

absolute; for instance many pathogens which initially grow between host cells may subsequently enter the cells once these become moribund.

Intercellular relationships are characteristic of relatively unspecialized pathogens which grow between cell walls and in intercellular spaces. Host cells are often killed in advance of invasion, through the action of enzymes or toxins produced by the pathogen. It seems unlikely that these necrotrophic pathogens ever make direct contact with living host protoplasm, and even if they do the host–pathogen interface is relatively short-lived. In contrast, intracellular relationships involve a more permanent contact between the partners, and penetrated host cells may remain apparently healthy for an extended period of time.

Structure and function of haustoria

In the majority of biotrophic fungi, haustoria develop from intercellular hyphae, branches of which are cut off by septa to form haustorial mother cells. The major part of the pathogen remains intercellular and the relationship is therefore intermediate between simple intercellular types and truly intracellular pathogens.

The process whereby haustoria penetrate host cells is rather similar to the way in which infection hyphae enter the epidermis; the host cell wall is breached by a narrow hypha which subsequently inflates within the lumen of the cell (Fig. 7.1i). In the powdery mildews the two processes are one and the same thing, as the pathogen only makes contact with the host via hausoria (Fig. 4.2). Where the haustorial neck passes through the cell wall, callose may be deposited in the form of a collar (Fig. 7.1iv). This is believed to be a host reaction, as callose deposits can frequently be observed forming on the inner face of the host cell wall prior to penetration. The developing hausorium then passes through this deposit which remains as a collar around the penetration site.

Although haustoria penetrate through the host cell wall, the plasma membrane remains intact as an invagination surrounding the haustorium. The interface between host and pathogen protoplasm is therefore a complex zone comprising the fungal membrane, the fungal cell wall and an extra-austorial membrane. In addition, there is often a distinct layer of amorhous material between the fungal cell wall and the extrahaustorial membrane (Fig. 7.1i). This matrix is sometimes described as the zone of apposition; its origin and biochemical nature is obscure, but it may represent a secretory response by the host. In some resistant hosts the haustorium is surrounded by an especially thick encasement or sheath which presumably seals it off and prevents the establishment of an effective parasitic relationship (Fig. 7.1ii). More precise characterization of these interfacial layers is now being attempted using chemical and enzymatic dissection methods in which different types of compound are specifically removed from the tissue section prior to microscopic examination.

Haustoria provide for an intimate contact between the pathogen and its host and increase the surface area available for exchange of materials. They are rich in mitochondria, ribosomes and vesicles, and thus seem to be sites of intense metabolic activity. Haustoria are presumed to function as organs of absorption but conclusive physiological data to support this view have proved difficult to obtain. Direct measurement of solute uptake by haustoria has been achieved only recently by isolating haustorial complexes from the epidermal cells of plants infected with powdery mildew fungi. Radioactively labelled carbon fed to the host as $^{14}CO_2$ is, as suspected, transferred into these haustoria. Using this technique it has also proved possible to measure the uptake of vital dyes or labelled sugars by the isolated haustorial complexes themselves. Results, while confirming that haustoria absorb photosynthetic products from the host, also suggest that the presence of host cytoplasm is essential for any nutrient uptake to occur.

Typically, host–pathogen interfaces involving haustoria are found in biotrophic fungi, such as the rusts and powdery mildews. In these relationships there are surprisingly few changes in the ultrastructure of penetrated host cells, at least during early stages of infection. Apparently normal chlorolasts and mitochondria are present, although the host cell nucleus may be swollen. It has often been reported that host cell organelles are clustered around haustoria (Fig. 7.1iii) but it is not clear whether this is a functional relationship or some artefact of the preparation of the material for electron microscopy. In later stages of infection there are visible changes in various cell organelles, such as the appearance of crystalline inclusions within microoodies. Many of these changes are superficially similar to the ultrastructural changes in senescent and virus-infected cells. Even so, some cells still appear to be viable long after penetration by pathogen haustoria. For example, in flax infected by the rust *Melampsora lini* there is little evidence of ultrastructural disorganization in cells containing haustoria up to two weeks after infection. Not all haustorial relationships are so benign. Haustoria are formed by *Phytophthora infestans* but penetrated cells quickly become necrotic. The relationship in this case is much more transitory.

Intracellular pathogens

Intracellular relationships are typical of some mutualistic associations, for example the root nodule bacterium *Rhizobium* and arbuscular mycorrhizas. In this context it is interesting to note the theory that the chloroplasts and mitochondria of eukaryotic cells may have arisen from endosymbiotic micro-organisms. A few pathogenic fungi also live inside host cells. The club-root pathogen exists in the form of a naked cell or PLASMODIUM, and the interface consists simply of the plasmodial cell membrane along with a second surrounding membrane which is believed to originate from the host. An even more intimate contact is found in parasitic chytrids such as *Olpidium*. Here the fungal cell is not surrounded by a host membrane and it is therefore in direct contact with the host cytoplasm.

A similar type of relationship has been found in cells infected by mycoplasmas, but the ultimate example of an intracellular pathogen is the virus. Virus particles occur within cytoplasm, nuclei and plastids. Because of their unique properties, viruses are not directly comparable to other pathogens in relation to interfacial characteristics. It is believed that successful replication of viruses depends upon a virus particle becoming adsorbed to specific cell receptor sites where removal of the coat protein takes place. It is not clear whether this essential step occurs at the cell membrane or within the cell, but either way the interface during multiplication is between a naked genome and the host protoplasm.

HOST REACTIONS TO PENETRATION

The initial events during host–pathogen interaction appear to be similar irrespective of whether the combination is compatible or incompatible (Fig. 3.1). Thus, in the case of a fungal pathogen penetrating a highly resistant host, spore germination, growth of the germ tube, appressorium formation and subsequent entry of the infection hypha all take place on a comparable time scale to these events on a host lacking resistance. At this early stage in the interaction it is often impossible to distinguish between the two host reaction types. Once the pathogen begins to breach the cell wall, however, events take a very different course depending upon the degree of host resistance. If the combination is compatible, further hyphal growth and invasion of host tissues continues unrestricted. In resistant hosts, however, a number of changes take place in penetrated cells and adjacent tissues which ultimately halt the advance of the pathogen.

Changes in host cell walls

The first detectable response of a plant cell to an invading micro-organism is often an alteration in the appearance or properties of the cell wall. For instance, attempted penetration of cereal leaves by non-pathogenic or avirulent fungi is accompanied by the deposition of a plug of material, known as a papilla, directly beneath the penetration site (Fig. 7.2). The epidermal cell wall surrounding the papilla may be changed to leave a disc-shaped zone or halo. Similar thickening and modification of host cell walls has been observed in other plant–fungus interactions; root cortical cells penetrated by root-infecting fungi may form characteristic protrusions of the wall known as lignitubers. Collectively, all these structures involving the accretion of new wall material are described as WALL APPOSITIONS.

Morphologically, wall deposits of various kinds appear similar, but what are they made of? Studies using histochemical stains or fluorescence microscopy have shown that quite different types of material accumulate, ranging from minerals such as silica to complex organic polymers like lignin. Table 7.2 lists some of the changes known to take place in response to infection.

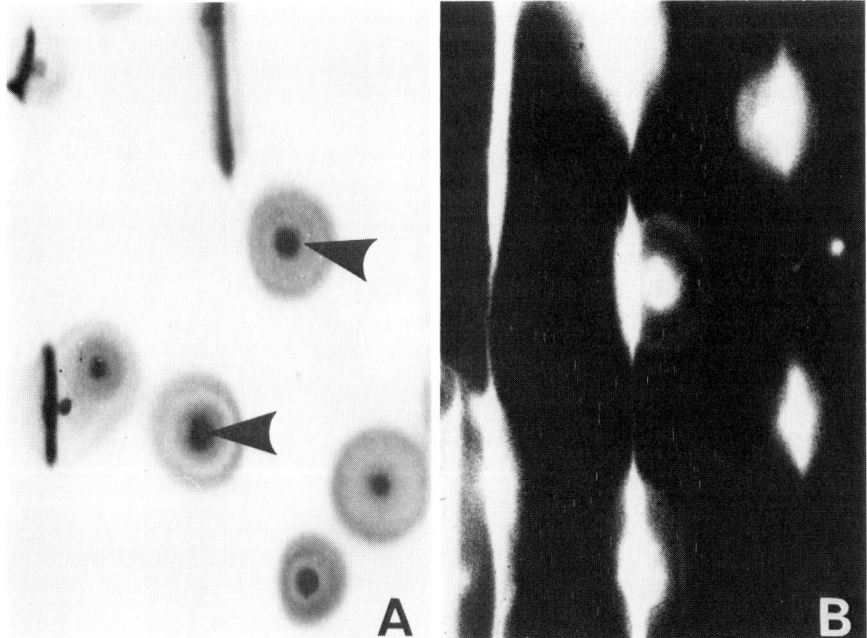

Figure 7.2 Epidermal strips taken from wheat leaves 24 h after inoculation with the fungus *Botrytis cinerea*. The stained preparation viewed by light microscopy (A) shows papillae and haloes at sites of attempted penetration (arrowed). Fluorescence microscopy (B) reveals autofluorescence at these sites and similar changes in adjacent lateral cell walls. (After Ride & Pearce, 1979.)

Although the accumulation of reaction material in cell walls is one of the earliest and most regular plant responses to challenge by a pathogen, there is debate about the importance of these structures in host resistance. The most obvious suggestion is that wall appositions impede penetration by the pathogen, either by increasing the strength and thickness of the cell wall or by enhancing its resistance to enzymic attack. Alternatively, successful parasitism may be impaired through changes in the permeability of cell walls. Finally it should be noted that the monomeric precursors of wall polymers, such as lignin, may themselves be toxic to micro-organisms. These various possibilities are listed in Table 7.3. What is not clear, however, is the extent to which any or all of these functions actually determine the outcome of a particular host–pathogen confrontation. Wall appositions are also produced in response to other types of injury, and it is

Table 7.2 Some cell wall changes in response to infection.

(1) Deposition of callose
(2) Deposition of suberin
(3) Impregnation with oxidized phenols, e.g. melanins
(4) Accumulation of calcium or silicon
(5) Lignification

Table 7.3 Possible functions of cell wall changes in host resistance.

(1) Mechanical barrier
(2) Increased resistance to cell-wall-degrading enzymes
(3) Reduced diffusion of compounds from host to pathogen or *vice versa*
(4) Direct toxicity of wall precursors, e.g. phenols, to pathogen

possible that they may be a non-specific wound response and therefore of secondary importance.

As we shall see in the next section, detecting host reactions to infection is comparatively easy, but proving a direct causal link between the observed cytological events and resistance is another matter.

The hypersensitive response

At the turn of the century, the American plant pathologist Marshall Ward, working on rust fungi infecting grasses, noted that in resistant hosts the cells adjacent to the infection site rapidly became discoloured, granular and necrotic. A few years later the term 'hypersensitive' was introduced to describe this type of reaction; host cells are apparently so sensitive to the pathogen that they collapse and die as soon as they are penetrated (Fig. 7.3).

The hypersensitive response has been the subject of intense study, partly because it is a clear example of the dynamic role of the host in the early stages of pathogen attack, but also because it confers a high degree of resistance on the host and has therefore tended to be the type of resistance

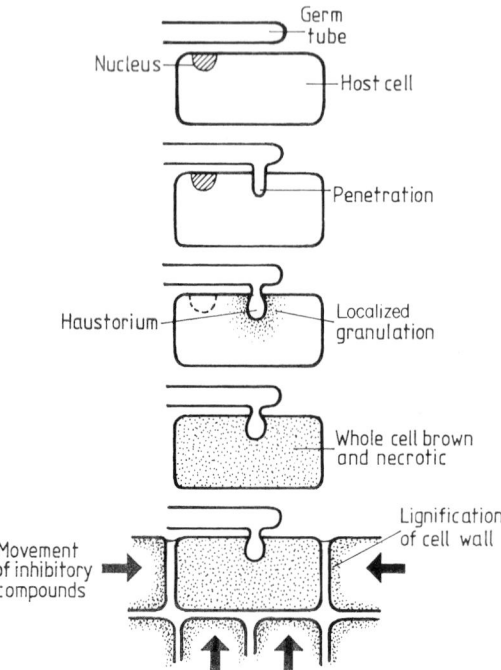

Figure 7.3 Diagrammatic sequence of events in the hypersensitive response of an epidermal cell.

selected for by the plant breeder. For instance, the resistance genes (R genes) introduced into the cultivated potato (*Solanum tuberosum*) through hybridization with the wild South American species *S. demissum* give good protection against specific races of *Phytophthora infestans*. Resistance controlled by these R genes is expressed as an hypersensitive response against incompatible races of the fungus. The high degree of specificity has proved in this case to be a stumbling block, as new races capable of overcoming the effects of these genes have arisen (see Chapter 10). Nevertheless, hypersensitivity has continued to attract interest, particularly now it is realized that this type of defence reaction is widespread amongst plants and effective against a variety of pathogens.

Initially, hypersensitivity was thought of as being significant only in interactions involving biotrophic fungi. Immediate death of the living cells would alone be sufficient to prevent the fungus from establishing an effective relationship. For a while this simple but attractive hypothesis seemed to be an adequate explanation for the basis of hypersensitive resistance. However, superficially similar and equally effective host reactions were found to occur with necrotrophic fungi and bacteria. In many respects the local lesion reaction of plants to viruses also bears similarities to an hypersensitive response; necrosis of cells around the inoculation site apparently prevents the virus from spreading systemically throughout the host.

The fact that hypersensitive resistance operates against both necrotrophs and biotrophs indicates that cell death may not in itself determine the fate of the pathogen. Instead it appears that host cell necrosis is accompanied by a whole series of events, including changes in oxidative metabolism, the accumulation of toxic compounds and the lignification of cell walls. The breakdown of membranes and the cellular disorganization that accompanies necrosis may in fact trigger metabolic changes in adjacent living cells. The sum total of these changes is the creation of an inhibitory environment which restricts further growth of the pathogen, either by starving it or poisoning it or physically walling it in or a combination of all three. The biochemical changes associated with hypersensitive-cell death will be discussed further in Chapter 8. For the moment we will concern ourselves with the cytological evidence, and the controversy surrounding hypersensitivity as a primary determinant of resistance.

The classical view of hypersensitivity

The original concept of hypersensitivity envisaged a straightforward sequence of events. During penetration, host cells swiftly die upon contact with the pathogen and the pathogen then ceases to grow. In effect, the host 'sacrifices' several cells so that the rest can survive. Let us return to the example of potato tissue containing a specific R gene. With a compatible race of the blight fungus, that is one able to overcome the effects of this gene, penetrated cells remain viable for up to 48 hours after initial contact

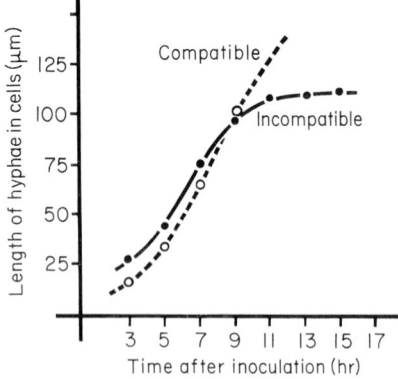

Figure 7.4 Total length of hyphae of compatible and incompatible races of *Phytophthora infestans* in potato cells. Incompatible cells die within 3 hours of inoculation while compatible cells are alive after 48 hours (data from Tomiyama, 1971).

with the pathogen. Similar cells penetrated by an incompatible race begin to degenerate within one hour of contact and die within two to three hours. Comparison of growth rates of compatible and incompatible races of the pathogen in cells of one cultivar has shown that there is very little difference between the two until at least eight hours after penetration (Fig. 7.4). In other words, the death of host cells precedes inhibition of pathogen growth by several hours. This observation is consistent with the classical view of hypersensitivity, i.e. the critical factor restricting the pathogen is the speed at which host cells die.

While the typical hypersensitive response is usually visualized as involving one or at the most a few host cells, in reality a gradation of reaction types exhibited. Figure 7.5 shows the reaction of an oilseed rape cultivar to infection by the downy mildew fungus *Peronospora parasitica*. The first few cells penetrated by fungal haustoria around each infection site have become necrotic, and the pathogen is contained. In a fully susceptible host, the fungus grows extensively throughout the mesophyll tissues without inducing necrosis of host cells. Between these two extremes there are cultivars which exhibit intermediate reactions, with corresponding variations in the extent of colonization and the amount of necrosis. In some cases, the pathogen continues to grow even though many of the penetrated cells appear dead. These subtle distinctions between reaction types may be a question of differences in the timing of cell death and associated biochemical events. One should also note that the reaction type may be radically altered by environmental conditions.

Is hypersensitivity important?

The view that hypersensitivity is a primary determinant of resistance in incompatible host–pathogen combinations has recently been questioned. When wheat leaves possessing hypersensitive resistance towards specific races of *Puccinia graminis* var. *tritici* are detached from the host plant their resistance is lowered. The host reaction type is, in effect, altered from

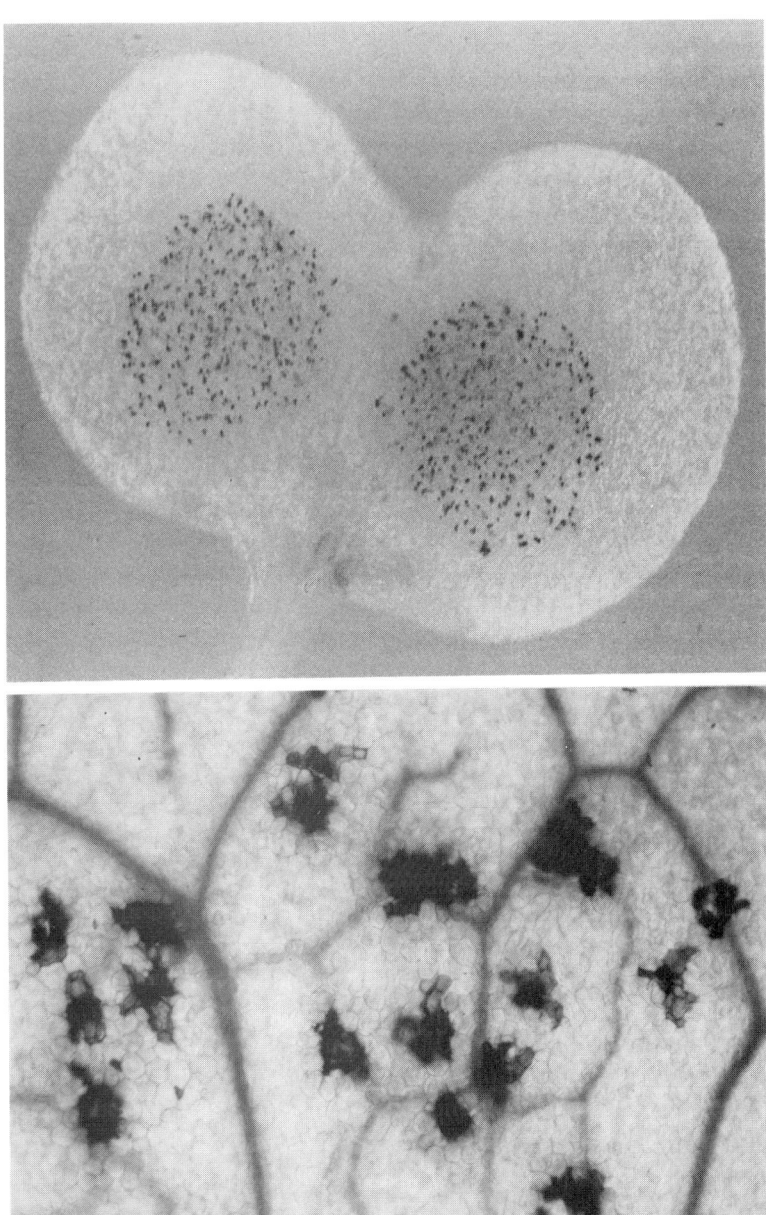

Figure 7.5 Restriction of pathogen development and hypersensitive-cell death. In the upper photograph the macroscopic response of a *Brassica* cotyledon to two drops of inoculum containing *Peronospora parasitica* sporangia shows as a large number of small, discrete, necrotic lesions. The extent of each lesion can be judged more exactly in the lower photograph, in which the host response to individual penetration hyphae is seen. The pathogen's infection hypha is in every instance contained within a small group of dark-coloured cells which are probably necrotic.

incompatible to compatible. In spite of this reduction in resistance, an apparently normal hypersensitive response still occurs. The inference here is that the development of the pathogen is determined independently of hypersensitive cell death. Other studies on the relationship between pathogen growth rates and host cell necrosis in cereals resistant to rust fungi have indicated that fungal growth is slowed down prior to cell penetration. This is at variance with the potato late blight example discussed above, and also with data from some imcompatible host–downy-mildew combinations.

Further support for the view that hypersensitivity is incidental to the processes controlling the outcome of the host–pathogen interaction has come from studies using inhibitors, such as antibiotics. If one treats a compatible potato–*Phytophthora* combination with the antibiotic streptomycin it is possible to induce an hypersensitive response. This conversion of a compatible reaction into an hypersensitive response can be interpreted as evidence that the fate of the pathogen is decided prior to host cell death. Presumably the antibiotic alters the normal time sequence of infection by slowing down or halting growth of the pathogen; in the absence of inhibition the fungus is able to grow quickly into further cells beyond the infection court. A further implication is that the antibiotic damages the pathogen, and as a result some product or products released by the dying pathogen trigger off the hypersensitive response. In naturally occurring hypersensitive responses some factor might initially inhibit the pathogen, thereby initiating the whole sequence of events. According to this explanation, hypersensitivity is a consequence, rather than a cause, of resistance. This theory is not, however, consistent with all the facts and there is still debate as to the real significance of these results.

Figure 7.6 summarizes two possible sequences of events involved in the hypersensitive response.

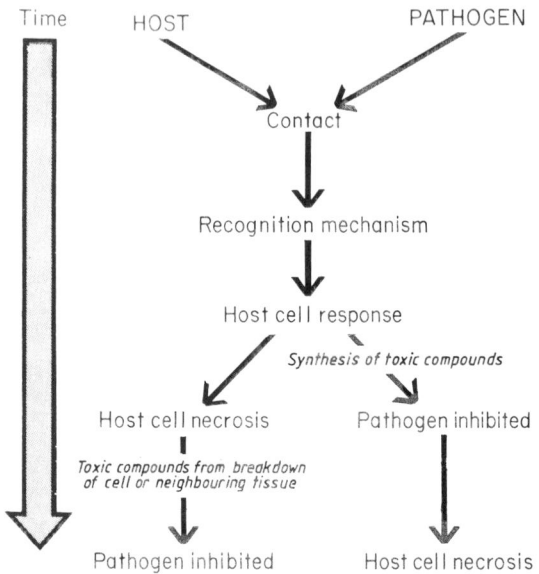

Figure 7.6 Two possible pathways of the hypersensitive response.

The hypersensitive reaction of plants to bacteria and viruses seems to be similar to that towards fungi inasmuch as it also involves cell necrosis and the accumulation of inhibitory compounds. However, unlike fungi, bacteria do not directly penetrate host cells, and are generally confined to intercellular spaces. Experiments usually entail infiltration of host leaves with large numbers of bacteria. Correspondingly, this results in extensive tissue necrosis and the formation of a lesion within which bacterial multiplication is restricted. The local lesion type of reaction to viruses also results in fairly extensive necrotic areas.

Just as there is debate about the role of hypersensitivity in resistance to fungi, so the extent to which host cell necrosis limits the spread of viruses is also a matter of controversy. Infective virus particles have been isolated from cells beyond the necrotic area, and virus localization probably occurs in cells around the margin of the lesion rather than in the lesion itself. If this is the case then necrosis is a secondary phenomenon.

Summary

We have devoted a comparatively large amount of space to a discussion of hypersensitivity, partly because it remains a controversial topic, but also because it embraces a number of cytological and biochemical changes relevant to active defence mechanisms in general. Undoubtedly, much of the dispute over the significance of hypersensitivity has arisen from a tendency to regard all defence reactions involving cell death as being identical. It is quite possible, however, that the precise sequence of events may be unique to each particular host–pathogen combination.

The broad similarities in the cellular reactions of plants to a range of different pathogens have been interpreted as providing evidence that plants share a common resistance mechanism, analogous to the immune system of animals. Alternatively, the similarities might suggest that these reactions are merely stress responses and incidental to the mechanisms which determine host–pathogen specificity. This topic will be discussed further in Chapter 9.

POST-INFECTIONAL CHANGES IN HOST PHYSIOLOGY

The invasion of the host by a foreign organism leads, sooner or later, to changes in host physiology. If the organism is a pathogen, these changes will eventually prove deleterious to the host. Alternatively, where the pathogen fails to establish itself, these changes may be important in preventing the pathogen from gaining a foothold. In practice it is often difficult to distinguish between post-infectional changes which are linked with resistance processes, and those which are related to pathogenesis, that is, disease development. Plants infected by quite different types of pathogens often exhibit very similar physiological symptoms. These similarities at first sight suggest that plants possess a common pathway of response to infection. However, many of the physiological effects we are about to describe also result if plants are subject to other forms of stress, such as mechanical or chemical injury. It should be borne in mind that some of the gross changes in the physiology of diseased plants represent a non-specific response to cellular damage inflicted by physical, chemical or microbial agents. An analysis of post-infectional changes in host physiology may, nevertheless, help to elucidate the mechanisms by which plants resist pathogenic attack, or clarify the ways in which pathogens cause disease.

Respiration

As parasitism involves a nutritional relationship much of the work on the physiology of infected plants has been concerned with energy metabolism. One of the most prominent features of diseased plants is a substantial increase in respiration rate. This is equally true for diseases involving fungi, bacteria and viruses, although most of the available information has been obtained from plants infected by biotrophic fungi. Figure 7.7 shows the rate of oxygen uptake in cabbage cotyledons during colonization by *Peronospora parasitica*. A similar pattern is seen in plants infected by rusts or powdery mildews. The increase in respiration rate commences at the onset of the first visible symptoms and rises to a peak coincident with the sporulation of the pathogen. This inevitably raises the question as to whether the increase is simply due to the additional respiration of the pathogen itself, rather than to a genuine host response. This, like many other apparently simple questions in host–pathogen physiology, is not easy to answer. Several lines of evidence suggest that while the pathogen makes some contribution to the increase, the greater part of it cannot be explained on this basis.

Powdery mildew fungi are only in intimate contact with their host where the haustoria enter epidermal cells. It is possible to peel off the epiphytic mycelium of the pathogen and measure the respiration rate of the host leaf with only an insignificant portion of the fungus (viz. the haustoria) remaining. Experiments like this have shown that the increase in respiration is maintained even after removal of the pathogen. There are alternative ways

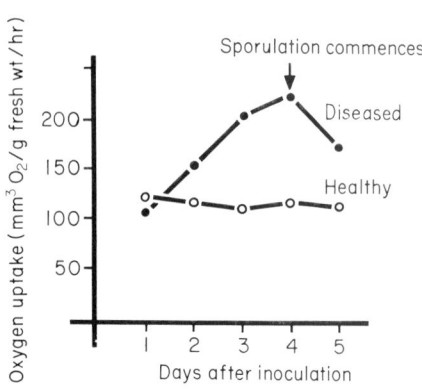

Figure 7.7 Oxygen uptake by healthy cabbage cotyledons and cotyledons affected by *Peronospora* (data from Thornton & Cooke, 1974).

of approaching this problem; for instance, one can measure the respiratory rate of uninfected tissues adjacent to lesions containing the pathogen or, in the case of facultative pathogens, one is able to examine the effects of toxic factors produced in culture on the respiratory metabolism of host cells. Using both approaches enhanced rates of host respiration have been found.

Perhaps the most convincing argument in support of the idea that increased post-infectional respiration is due to a stimulation of host metabolism comes, however, from studies on virus diseases. Viruses, being non-cellular, possess no respiratory apparatus of their own, and yet a similar stimulation of respiration rate is found in a variety of viral infections. For example, the development of necrotic local lesions in *Nicotiana glutinosa* inoculated with TMV is accompanied by a pronounced increase in respiration.

All in all, the rise in respiration rates following infection would seem mainly to represent a response by host tissues. This response bears similarities to the transitory increase in respiration observed in plants wounded by mechanical injury.

The mechanism of respiratory increase

Although measurements of the gross respiratory rate (in terms of either oxygen uptake or carbon dioxide evolution) indicate that the physiology of the host is altered by infection, this information is, in isolation, of limited value. It does not tell us anything about the mechanism of the increase, nor how the pathogen stimulates the host. Unfortunately, most of our present knowledge of disease physiology has not progressed much beyond this sort of 'tip of the iceberg' observation. There are, however, a number of theories which seek to explain the enhanced respiration rate in diseased plants (Fig. 7.8).

In healthy cells, respiration is regulated by a number of factors the most important of which is the availability of adenosine diphosphate (ADP). Agents such as 2,4-dinitrophenol (DNP) stimulate the respiration rate by 'uncoupling' electron transfer from oxidative phosphorylation. In essence, this means that while electron flow continues, the regeneration of adenosine triphosphate (ATP) from ADP and inorganic phosphate no longer takes place. Due to the continued consumption of ATP in cellular metabolism, the pool of ADP is replenished and the usual feedback mechanism based on the availability of ADP no longer operates.

It has been suggested that pathogens may uncouple host respiration ((a) in Fig. 7.8). This hypothesis is based on evidence that respiration in diseased tissues is no longer stimulated by treatment with DNP. In addition, the level of ATP is often lower in infected tissues. Presumably some compound produced by the pathogen acts as an uncoupler in host cells, but whatever the attractions of this hypothesis it has received little experimental support and recently several other explanations have gained ground.

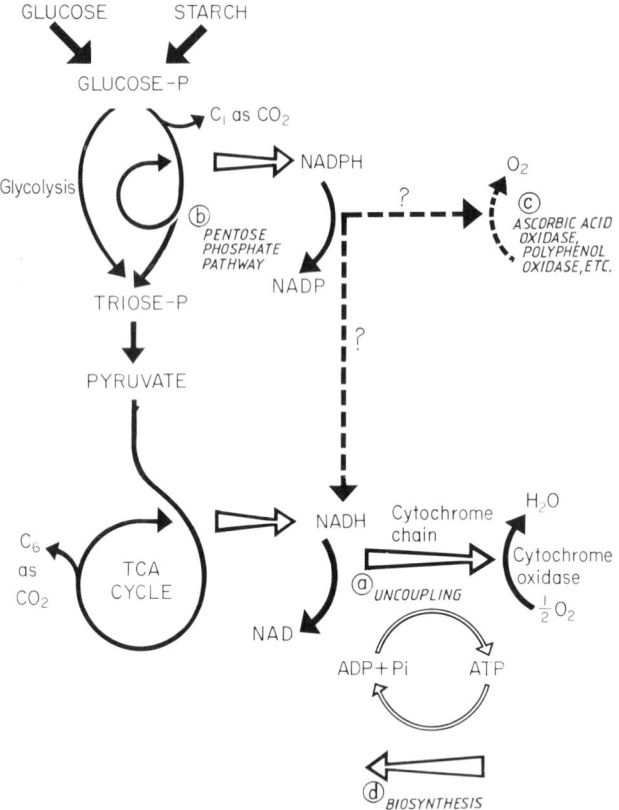

Figure 7.8 Theories concerning stimulation of respiration in infected plants. For comment on ⓐ – ⓓ see text on pp. 121–3.

The major metabolic pathway for the degradation of glucose to pyruvate is glycolysis, otherwise known as the Embden–Meyerhof pathway. An alternative route for the production of pyruvate, the pentose phosphate pathway, is generally considered to be of less importance although it does provide intermediates for the biosynthesis of many vital cellular materials, including nucleic acids. Assessment of the relative contribution of each pathway relies largely on data from labelling studies in which radioactive carbon is incorporated into either the C_6 or the C_1 position of the glucose molecule. Subsequent measurement of the ratio of labelled carbon dioxide released from each source during respiration indicates which pathway is predominant; activation of the pentose phosphate pathway leads to an increased contribution from the C_1 position, and hence lowers the C_6/C_1 ratio. In infected plants, the C_6/C_1 ratio is typically lower than the values obtained from healthy tissues, suggesting that there is increased participation of the pentose route (ⓑ in Fig. 7.8). Assays of several pentose phosphate pathway enzymes support this idea, their activity being higher in diseased tissues. It should be borne in mind, however, that most of the available data have been obtained from host–pathogen systems involving fungi. The pentose phosphate pathway operates at a higher level in fungi than in higher plants, and the increased contribution in infected tissues may simply reflect this feature of fungal metabolism.

Alterations in the pathway of glucose degradation would not necessarily result in a rise in gross respiration rate, although the pentose phosphate pathway is marginally less efficient in generating ATP. It now seems likely that the real significance of the switch to the pentose pathway is linked to its role in the biosynthesis of various compounds. As well as providing pentoses for the biosynthesis of nucleic acids, pentose phosphate intermediates are involved in the production of numerous aromatic compounds, notably phenols and their derivatives. Many of these compounds are associated with host defence reactions, a topic which will be discussed further in Chapter 8.

In addition to changes in respiratory pathways, alternative terminal oxidation systems may operate in diseased tissues (ⓒ in Fig. 7.8). Apart from the usual cytochrome system terminating with cytochrome oxidase, systems involving phenol oxidases and ascorbic acid oxidase have been detected in plants. Both of these enzymes appear to be activated in diseased tissues. The precise mechanism and significance of such oxidation systems is not clear, but phenol oxidases play a part in the production of phenolic compounds, an observation consistent with the general pattern of post-infectional metabolism. It also seems likely that the reduced coenzyme NADPH generated by the pentose pathway is oxidized by one of these enzymes, rather than by the cytochrome system. As far as is known, these alternative oxidases are unable to participate in the formation of ATP during oxygen uptake.

Although evidence exists in support of each of the above theories regarding respiratory changes in the infected host, the most satisfactory explanation for the increased rate of metabolism in infected plants is perhaps the most obvious. With biotrophic pathogens the increased respiration is associated with enhanced synthetic, rather than degradative, metabolism; in other words, there is a general increase in the biosynthetic activities of the host (ⓓ in Fig. 7.8). This increase in turn requires more rapid utilization of ATP and thereby removes the restraints imposed by the availability of ADP. It is significant that in many diseases caused by fungi the major increase in respiration coincides with the onset of sporulation by the pathogen. This is precisely the time when the fungus will be exerting the maximum drain on host nutrients due to the considerable energy input associated with the production of spores or other propagules. The biosynthesis of defence compounds by the host will also consume energy in the form of ATP.

In conclusion, an increase in host respiration, which in turn implies a general stimulation of host metabolism, is one of the most prominent physiological consequences of infection by pathogens. The basis for this stimulation presumably resides in increased activity of host enzymes, either through activation or the derepression of host genes. The molecular basis of these changes, and the pathogen-produced factors which may induce them, will be considered in Chapter 8.

Photosynthesis

Photosynthesis is the most distinctive physiological activity of green plants. The capture of solar energy by chlorophyll and its subsequent utilization to fix carbon dioxide into organic compounds is the basis of life on this planet. However, in spite of its fundamental importance, comparatively little is known about the effects of pathogens on photosynthesis.

Any pathogen which attacks green aerial tissues is likely to affect crop yield. In many cases the harmful effects of a pathogen can be directly attributed to the destruction of photosynthetic tissues. A serious outbreak of potato blight can completely defoliate an entire field while *Botrytis fabae* can cause necrotic patches which occupy over 50% of the leaf area of broad beans.

It is therefore obvious that one major result of pathogen invasion is a reduction in the photosynthetic capacity of a plant through the destruction of green tissue.

However, this simple conclusion ignores the possibility that there are effects in adjacent uninfected tissues and it tells us nothing about any changes in the photosynthetic process itself. For instance, with the example above, *Botrytis* on beans, measurement of the relative growth rate of infected plants has shown that it is similar to the growth rate of uninfected plants, even when 30–40% of the leaf area is removed. The implication here is that the photosynthetic efficiency of the remaining leaf tissue is enhanced to compensate for the loss in area. However, there is eventually an effect on yield, which in this case is due to a reduction in the number of pods formed per plant.

Chlorosis is one of the most common symptoms of plant disease. It is indicative of a reduction in the chlorophyll content of green tissues. A reduced chlorophyll content could be due either to the breakdown of chlorophyll or to the inhibition of chlorophyll synthesis. In chlorosis associated with virus infections, higher levels of the enzyme chlorophyllase have been detected, suggesting that chlorophyll is being degraded by the enzymic reaction:

$$\text{Chlorophyll} \xrightarrow{\text{Chlorophyllase}} \text{Chlorophyllide} + \text{Phytol}$$

In leaves infected by biotrophic fungi there is also a progressive loss in overall photosynthetic activity, although this is usually only noticeable in the later stages of infection, when premature senescence of the leaf may set in. Figure 7.9 shows the net photosynthetic rate of oak leaves infected by the powdery mildew pathogen *Microsphaera alphitoides*. There is a slight initial stimulation of photosynthesis in inoculated leaves, but this is followed

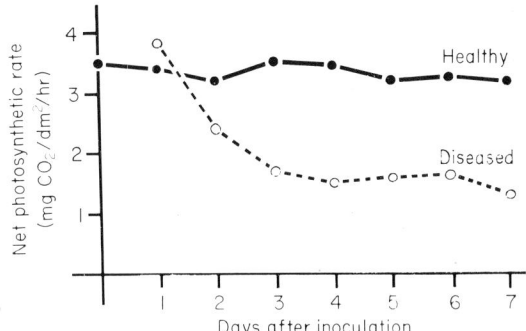

Figure 7.9 Changes in photosynthesis of oak leaves following infection by the powdery mildew fungus *Microsphaera alphitoides* (data from Hewitt & Ayres, 1975).

by a rapid decline. The rate of $^{14}CO_2$ uptake by leaf discs from sugar beet infected by powdery mildew is also reduced compared with healthy tissues (Fig. 7.10). Chloroplasts isolated from mildewed beet leaves show a reduced capacity to form ATP by non-cyclic photophosphorylation. In diseases caused by rust fungi, electron-microscope studies have shown that chloroplast ultrastructure is altered in the later stages of infection. Plastid membranes break down and the overall changes bear similarities to those seen in senescent cells.

Although the general pattern of photosynthesis in infected plants seems to involve a reduction in activity, there are exceptions. In uninfected bean leaves on plants infected by *Uromyces phaseoli*, fixation of radioactive carbon dioxide is actually stimulated compared with healthy controls (Fig. 7.11). This result is of particular interest as it demonstrates that post-infectional changes in photosynthesis may occur at a distance from the infection site.

The most important exception to the usual sequence of chlorosis and reduced photosynthetic activity is also seen in diseases caused by the rust fungi. This is the so-called 'green island' effect, where tissues in the vicinity of fungal pustules are green even though the surrounding areas of the leaf are chlorotic. There has been much discussion of the significance of these green islands because the selective retention of chlorophyll around infection

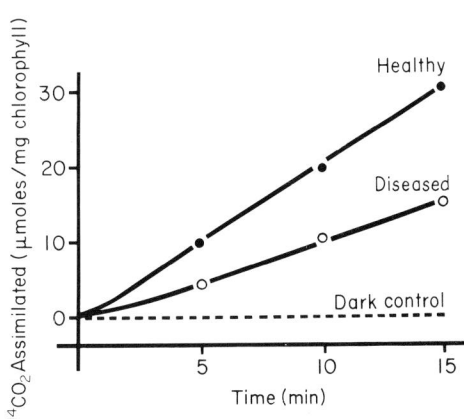

Figure 7.10 Effect of *Erysiphe polygoni* on the rate of photosynthetic $^{14}CO_2$ assimilation by sugar beet leaf discs (data from Magyarosy *et al.*, 1976).

125

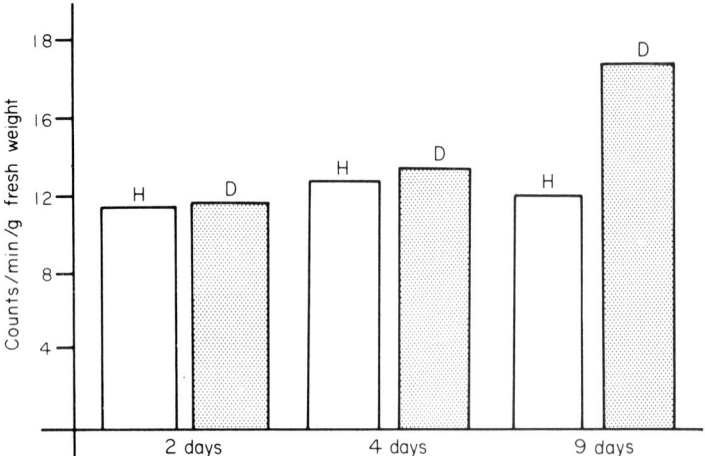

Figure 7.11 Comparison of $^{14}CO_2$ uptake by rust-free leaves from healthy (H) and rust-affected (D) bean plants at different times after inoculation (data from Livne, 1964).

sites suggests that the pathogen exerts some degree of control over host physiology. The similarities between this delay in senescence and the effects of hormonal factors, such as cytokinins, has prompted the view that the pathogen secretes hormonally active compounds. In diseases caused by powdery mildew fungi, evidence suggests that chlorophyll is initially degraded but subsequently resynthesized in areas of the leaf adjacent to disease lesions. Green islands are probably associated with the redirection of host nutrients which occurs in diseases caused by biotrophic parasites. Necrotrophic pathogens are generally less subtle in their effects and rapidly break down host organelles such as chloroplasts.

Translocation of nutrients and water

The damage caused by biotrophic pathogens is due, to some extent at least, to their ability to redirect host nutrients to their own ends. The idea that fungal colonies act as 'metabolic sinks' in their hosts is supported by radioisotope tracer experiments in which labelled carbon accumulates preferentially in disease lesions (Fig. 7.12). In this way, photosynthate originally destined for developing host tissues, such as new shoots or roots, is instead utilized by the pathogen. The reduced root growth and grain yield of cereals infected by rusts and powdery mildews is due to this disturbance in the nutrient balance of the plant. As is shown in Fig. 7.12, a large part of the imbalance seems to be caused by the retention of sugars and amino acids in the infected older leaves. Tracer experiments have also shown that carbon originally present in host sugars, such as sucrose, can be detected in typical fungal metabolites like the sugar alcohols, mannitol and arabitol. Although it is clear that host nutrients are taken up by the pathogen, the nature of the compounds which move from host to the pathogen is at present unresolved.

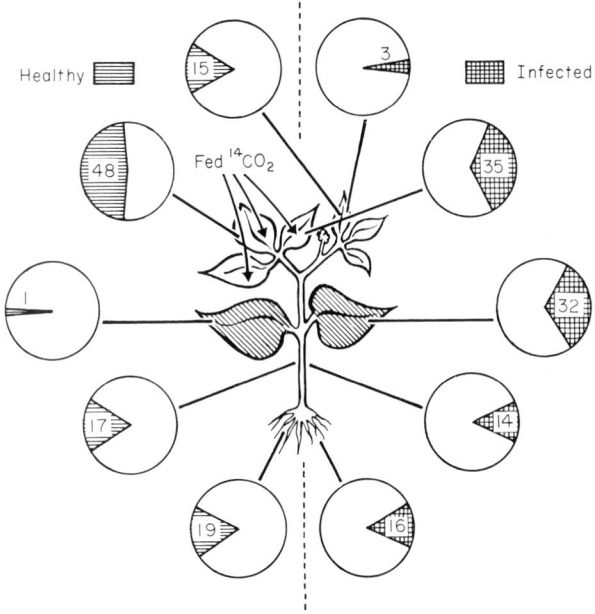

Figure 7.12 Translocation of ^{14}C in healthy bean plants and bean plants affected by *Uromyces phaseoli* after feeding $^{14}CO_2$ to healthy trifoliate leaves. Shading indicates sites of rust on unifoliate leaves of infected plants and numbers indicate percentage of total radioisotope in each organ (data from Livne & Daly, 1966).

The conversion of host sugars to fungal carbohydrates could in fact serve to maintain a concentration gradient and ensure a continued flow from host to fungus. Mobilization of storage polysaccharides, such as starch, can also occur. Cells penetrated by fungal haustoria often appear to contain fewer starch granules but accumulation of starch in tissues adjacent to disease lesions has also been reported.

The multiplication of viruses in plant cells is entirely at the expense of the host. Sequestration of host metabolites to make more virus particles may explain some of the deleterious effects of virus infection. In severe infections the virus particles themselves may come to represent about 10% of the dry weight of leaf tissues, and multiplication on this scale must severely tax the synthetic capacities of the host, particularly if the plant is growing under suboptimal conditions. Virus replication requires the synthesis of two components, nucleic acid and coat protein, and one major side effect of infection may therefore be a deficiency of inorganic nutrients, in particular phosphorus and nitrogen, available to the host.

The nutrient stress imposed by a redirection of host nutrients to satisfy the energy and biosynthetic needs of the pathogen is very different from that caused by pathogens which actually colonize the transporting tissues of the plant. Vascular wilt pathogens impair the flow of water and mineral salts through the xylem. Translocation of sugars through phloem tissues is also disrupted by some pathogens; a number of virus infections cause necrosis of phloem elements, resulting in nutrient imbalances in the host. For instance, potato plants infected by leafroll virus have higher than normal carbohydrate levels in their leaves, while that of the tubers is reduced. Two possible explanations of this symptom are reduced translocation of sugars due either to the inhibition of the process itself or to the breakdown of the phloem tissue. High concentrations of spiroplasmas often build up in the phloem elements of diseased plants but in this case symptoms, such as wilting and stunting, are thought to be due to production of a diffusible toxin rather than to occlusion of the vascular elements.

The interdependence of physiological processes such as ion uptake and the translocation of water and nutrients should be emphasized. In take-all disease of cereals, invasion of the root cortex by the pathogen does not significantly affect ion uptake or translocation. Instead the crucial stage appears to be the subsequent colonization of phloem tissues by the fungus. This reduces the translocation of nutrients to the apical meristems, with the result that the distal portions of the root cease to function and ion uptake is impaired.

The wilt syndrome

The most pronounced effect of vascular wilt pathogens is on the water economy of the host. In tomatoes infected by *Fusarium oxysporum* f.sp. *lycopersici* the resistance to water flow through the xylem is substantially increased compared to the resistance of uninfected stems. This effect can be partially explained on the basis of physical obstruction of the vessels by hyphae, but the vascular wilt syndrome is a great deal more complex than this. It involves host responses to infection as well as the pathogen and its products (Fig. 7.13). Blockages caused by the growth of the pathogen are compounded by its secretion of polysaccharides and pectolytic enzymes; in turn the host responds by producing gums and mucilages and by forming tyloses in the vessels. The end result is that water flow may be reduced to less than five per cent of that in healthy plants. As well as causing severe water stress, infection by wilt pathogens also reduces the passage of essential mineral ions to the leaves. The overall consequences of vascular blockage are, however, difficult to assess, as these pathogens also secrete toxins which have physiological effects throughout the plant.

Transpiration

Wilting is one of the most common disease symptoms in plants, but the physiological basis of the symptom is not the same in all cases. The water economy can be disrupted through reduced water uptake, reduced translocation or increased water loss through transpiration. Root-rot pathogens destroy root tissues, and therefore reduce the surface area available for uptake and disrupt the transport of water through the root system. The vascular wilt fungi reduce translocation and at the same time reduce the

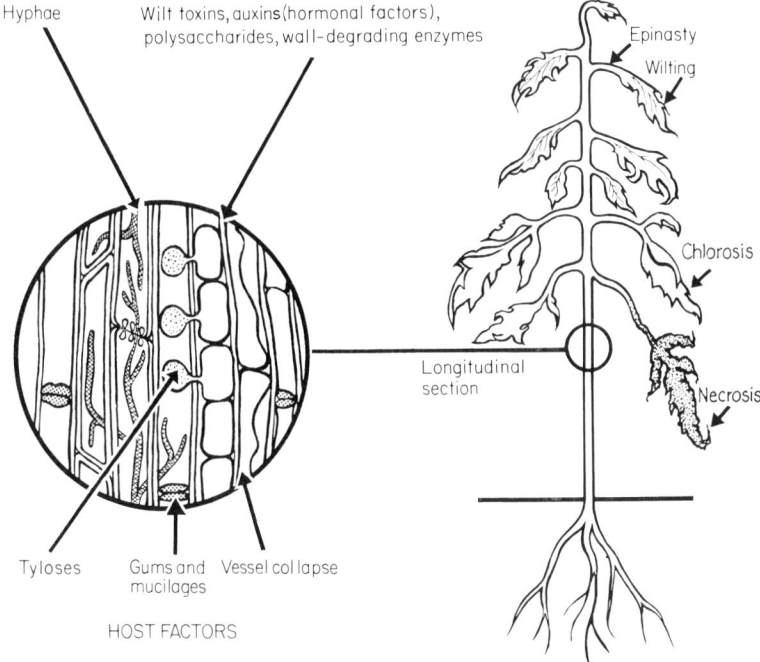

PATHOGEN FACTORS

Hyphae

Wilt toxins, auxins (hormonal factors),
polysaccharides, wall-degrading enzymes

Epinasty

Wilting

Chlorosis

Longitudinal
section

Necrosis

Tyloses

Gums and Vessel collapse
mucilages

HOST FACTORS

Figure 7.13 The vascular wilt syndrome. Wilting cannot be ascribed to any one factor.

transpiration rate. This second effect can be explained on the basis of water stress in the leaves, coupled with stomatal closure. Many other pathogens increase the transpiration rate (Fig. 7.14). This effect is predictable inasmuch as any pathogen which damages the surface layers of the leaf will increase cuticular transpiration and this may, in fact, be the major source of

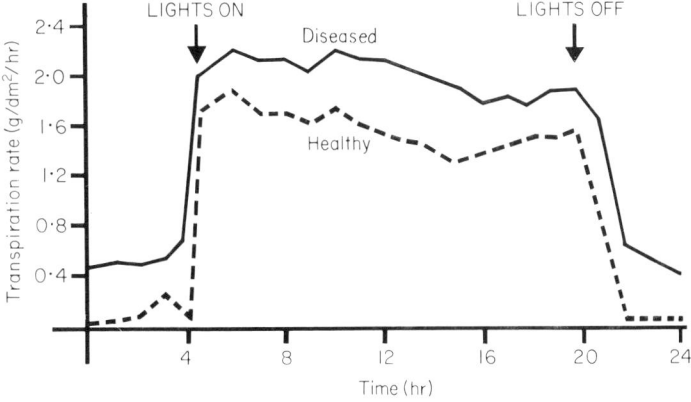

Figure 7.14 Transpiration rates over 24 hours of healthy barley plants (- - -) and barley plants affected by *Rhynchosporium secalis* (———). Arrows indicate duration of photoperiod. (Data from Ayres & Jones, 1975.)

129

the increased rate of water loss. Damage of this sort is often restricted to the reproductive phase of the pathogen's life cycle; the rust fungi form erumpent pustules which tear through the host epidermis prior to release of the spores (Fig. 5.8). At this point wilting often occurs for the first time. The physical damage inflicted on the host during sporulation is a good example of the indirect and harmful effects that biotrophic fungi have on the plant.

It is often difficult, however, to assess the basic reasons for increased transpiration in diseased plants. The data shown in Fig. 7.14 are from a relatively early stage of barley infection by *Rhynchosporium* when the host cuticle is still intact. A complicating factor is the stomatal behaviour of infected leaves. In the above example, a higher proportion of stomata remain open in the dark in infected plants, which no doubt contributes to the increased level of water loss. Abnormal opening of stomata also occurs in potato leaves infected by *Phytophthora infestans* (Fig. 7.15). Here the

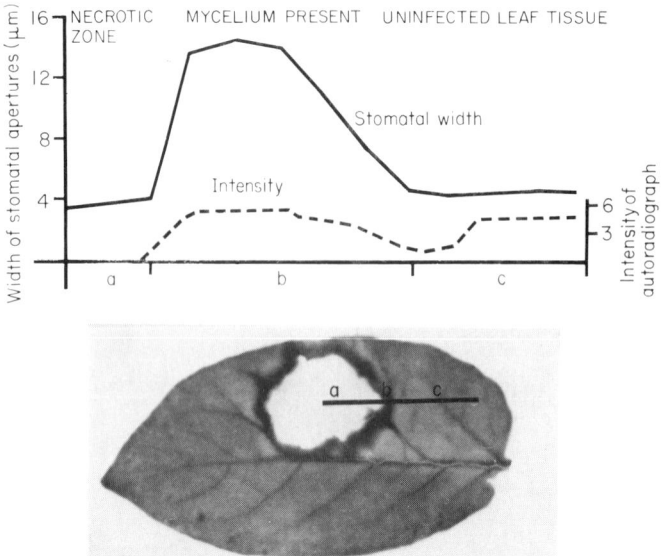

Figure 7.15 Stomatal width and corresponding uptake of $^{14}CO_2$ (measured as intensity of blackening on autoradiograph as below) in serial zones across the margin of a blight lesion on a potato leaf (data from Farrell *et al.*, 1969).

effect is confined to a zone surrounding the necrotic lesions. Stomata within this zone open abnormally wide and remain open in the dark; they therefore do not present an obstacle to the developing fungal sporangiophores, which characteristically emerge through the stomata at night. The physiological consequences of this alteration in stomatal behaviour are of particular interest. Fixation of $^{14}CO_2$ is enhanced in the same zone (Fig. 7.15), and a causal relationship between increased photosynthesis and higher rates of gas exchange through the open stomata has been suggested.

The few studies which have been made on the water relations of virus infected plants indicate that the transpiration rate is reduced, and the total water content of the host is lower. This is especially true in advanced infections.

Cell water relations

In addition to effects on the water economy of the whole plant, pathogens may also influence the water relations of individual cells. It is generally accepted that cell water relations are controlled by the plasma membrane, although in plant cells the rigid wall is also important in maintaining turgor. Due to its semipermeable properties, however, the plasma membrane is of central importance in regulating the passage of ions and organic molecules into and out of the cell. This membrane is a complex and dynamic structure which exerts a substantial degree of control over the movement of materials and thereby maintains a suitable intracellular environment for metabolism.

It has been known for some time that one of the most common effects of pathogens on plant cells is to increase their permeability. The membrane apparently loses its semipermeable properties and mineral ions and other

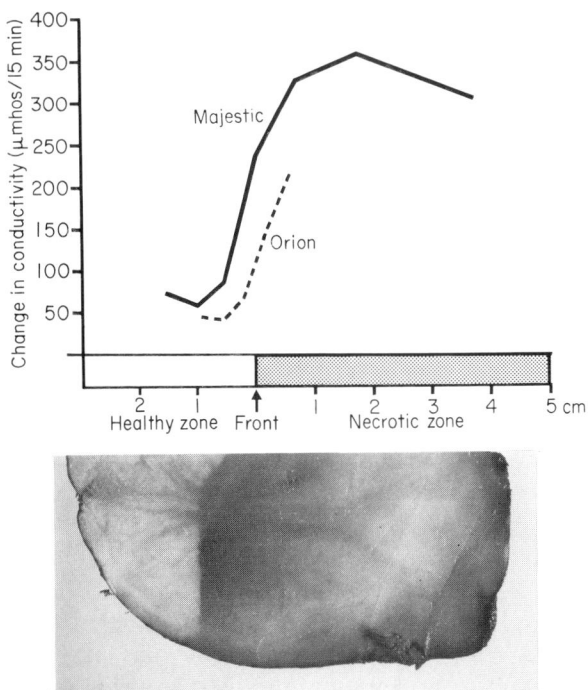

Figure 7.16 Effect of *Phytophthora erythroseptica* on electrolyte leakage from potato tubers cv Majestic and cv Orion. Arrow indicates advancing edge of necrotic lesion seen in the photograph below of a tuber cv Orion showing a typical pink-rot lesion. (data from Lucas, unpublished.)

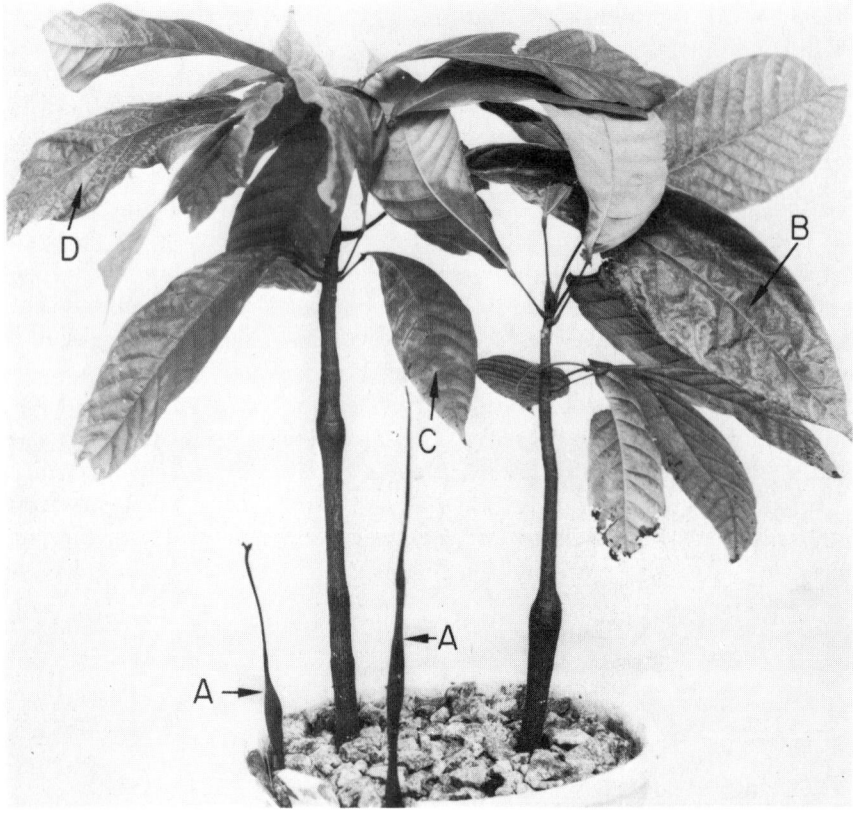

Figure 7.17 (i)   Cocoa plants, cultivar Amelonado, infected with cocoa swollen shoot virus. Nodal swellings (A) are associated with apical dieback. Leaf symptoms include vein clearing (B), vein banding (C) and fern-pattern (D). (Photograph by J.T. Legg.)

electrolytes leak out into the external medium. This effect is pronounced in soft-rot diseases caused by necrotrophic pathogens, in which host cell necrosis is a major feature (Fig. 7.16). In itself this observation is not very instructive as membrane disintegration would be expected to take place anyway in moribund or dead cells. What is of greater interest in these diseases is the actual cause of membrane damage (see Chapter 8).

It has been shown that biotrophic pathogens also increase the permeability of host tissues. Electron micrographs of haustoria indicate that the host plasma membrane around them is intact, but it sometimes appears to be altered structurally or chemically in comparison with healthy cell membranes. Cells penetrated by haustoria can still be plasmolysed, so the integrity of the host membrane is maintained. Nevertheless there is a definite increase in leakage of electrolytes from infected tissues, and it has been suggested that this change in the semipermeable properties of the plasma membrane is related to the uptake of nutrients by the pathogen. The redirection of host metabolism imposed by biotrophic fungi may well include subtle effects on host membranes, although the cells remain viable. Leakage

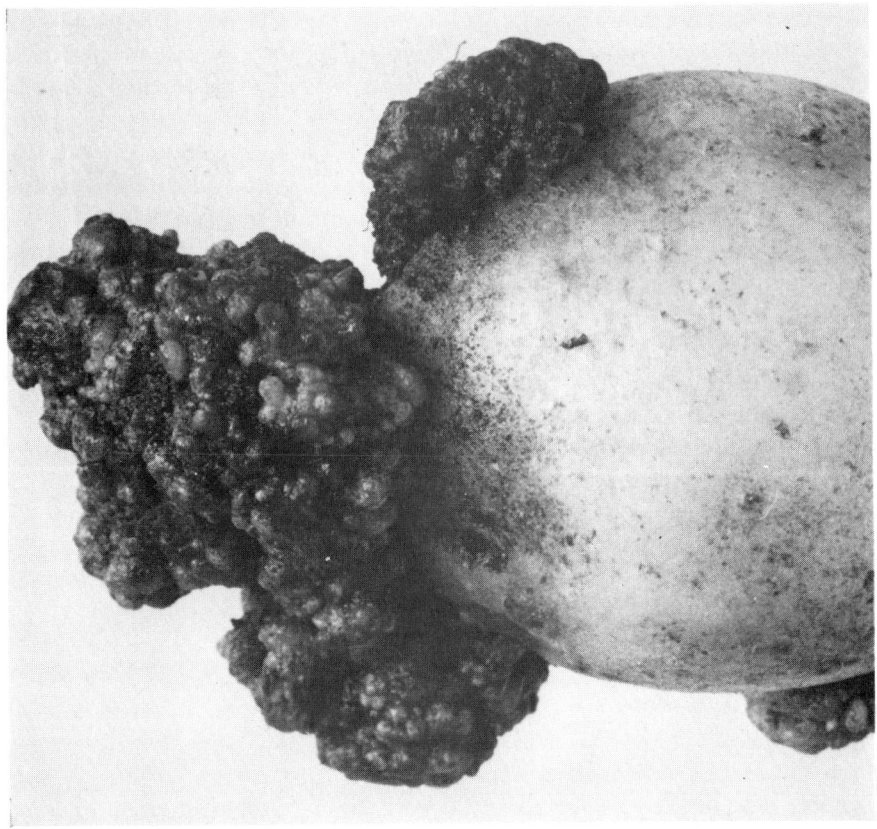

Figure 7.17 (ii) Potato tuber infected with *Synchytrium endobioticum*. The wart-like excrescences on the tuber are caused by cell division and cell enlargement following infection with the pathogen. (Photograph Crown Copyright.)

of electrolytes has also been recorded in virus-infected tissues, especially roots, but this does not seem to be a common symptom in these diseases.

The importance of membrane systems in the regulation of cell metabolism has only recently been fully appreciated. It is not surprising, therefore, that the effects of pathogens on cell membranes is currently a topic of major interest to plant pathologists. In addition to the plasma membrane itself, the cell also contains membrane-bound organelles, such as plastids, mitochondria, peroxisomes and lysosomes, and alterations in one or several of these type of organelle may be involved in many aspects of disease physiology.

Growth regulation

All plant pathogens affect the growth and development of their hosts to a greater or lesser extent. The diversion of nutrients or the destruction of host tissues will inevitably lead to reduced performance, and in some cases may severely stunt the plant. These effects on plant growth are, however, essentially indirect and therefore different from the specific growth abnormalities induced by a variety of pathogens. Symptoms such as galls and tumours, excessive branching, leaf epinasty, abnormal induction of adventitious roots and premature leaf abscission are all associated with changes in the control of plant growth and differentiation. Such deranged growth is characteristic of many diseases involving fungi, bacteria and viruses (Fig. 7.17).

Although plant morphogenesis is influenced by environmental conditions, control of the basic processes of cell division and differentiation is mediated by hormonal compounds such as indoleacetic acid, gibberellins, cytokinins and ethylene. Changes in the concentration or distribution of these hormones have widespread effects on the physiology of the plant. Because alterations in growth regulation can be attributed to hormonal changes, discussion of diseases involving growth abnormalities will be deferred until the next chapter.

Conclusion

It should be apparent from this review that many of the measurable changes in the physiology of infected plants are common to a variety of diseases. In the search for a unifying concept in host–pathogen interaction it is tempting to interpret these similarities as evidence for a common pathway or sequence of biochemical events following infection. Many of these gross alterations however, e.g. increased respiration and permeability changes, are also characteristic of plants damaged by non-microbial agents. In view of this, the explanation of resistance and pathogenesis may in fact be more to do with changes unique to infected plants rather than these general responses to stress conditions. This explanation must ultimately be sought in terms of molecular events, and the preliminary progress which has been made towards this end is the subject of the next chapter.

FURTHER READING

General texts

FRIEND J. & THRELFALL D.R. eds (1976) *Biochemical Aspects of Plant–Parasite Relationships.* Academic Press, London.
    Proceedings of a conference dealing with a wide range of topics relevant to both Chapters 7 and 9.

HEITEFUSS R. & WILLIAMS P.H. eds (1976) *Encyclopedia of Plant Physiology*, Vol. IV., *Physiological Plant Pathology.* Springer Verlag, Berlin.
    An imaginative compendium of papers dealing with a wide range of topics in plant pathology.

MACE M.E., BELL A.A. & BECKMAN C.H. eds (1981) *Fungal Wilt Diseases of Plants.* Academic Press, New York.
    See contributions of R.J. Green, An overview; R. Hall & W.E. McHardry, Water relations; and G.F. Pegg, Biochemistry and physiology of pathogenesis.

Reviews and original articles

AIST J.R. & ISRAEL H.W. (1977) Papilla formation: timing and significance during penetration of barley coleoptiles by *Erysiphe graminis hordei*. *Phytopathology* **67**, 455–461.

BUSHNELL W.R. & GAY J. (1978) Accumulations of solutes in relation to the structure and function of haustoria in powdery mildews. In *The Powdery Mildews* (ed. Spencer D.M.), pp. 183–235. Academic Press, London.

HICKEY E.L. & COFFEY M.D. (1978) A cytochemical investigation of the host-parasite interface in *Pisum sativum* infected by the downy mildew fungus *Peronospora pisi*. *Protoplasma* **97**, 201–220.

INGRAM D.S. (1978) Cell death and resistance to biotrophs. *Annals of Applied Biology* **89**, 291–5.

KIRÁLY Z., BARNA B. & ÉRSEK T. (1972) Hypersensitivity as a consequence, not the cause, of plant resistance to infection. *Nature* (London) **239**, 456–8.

MacLEAN D.J., SARGENT J.A., TOMMERUP J.C. & INGRAM D.S. (1974) Hypersensitivity as the primary event in resistance to fungal parasites. *Nature* (London) **249**, 186–7.

RIDE J.P. (1978) The role of cell wall alterations in resistance to fungi. *Annals of Applied Biology* **89**, 302–6.

8 Host-pathogen interaction at the molecular level

> "We have little exact knowledge of the chemico-physiological processes in the life of the parasitic fungi because the symbiotic relation puts great complications and difficulties in the way of their precise investigation"
> DE BARY (1831–1888)

At this point let us reconsider the diagram of host–pathogen interaction which we drew in Chapter 1.

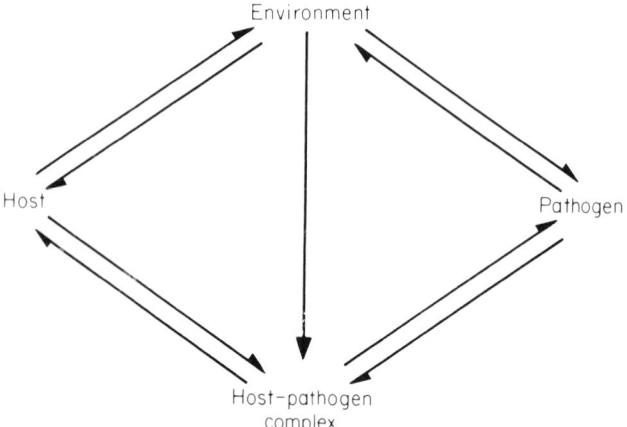

This scheme does not tell us anything about the kinds of interaction which take place within the host–pathogen complex itself. We should now draw a more detailed scheme which identifies some of these interactions (Fig. 8.1).

We have already considered the major part that environmental factors play in plant disease. Not only do they determine whether or not infection occurs, but they also influence disease development by their effects on host resistance and the growth rate of the pathogen.

Physical interactions are also important. These include features of the host, such as the cuticle, stomatal morphology and the endodermis, all of which can affect the host–pathogen relationship. In addition, one should recall that the physical damage inflicted on the host by the growth and reproduction of the pathogen is often a significant source of disease

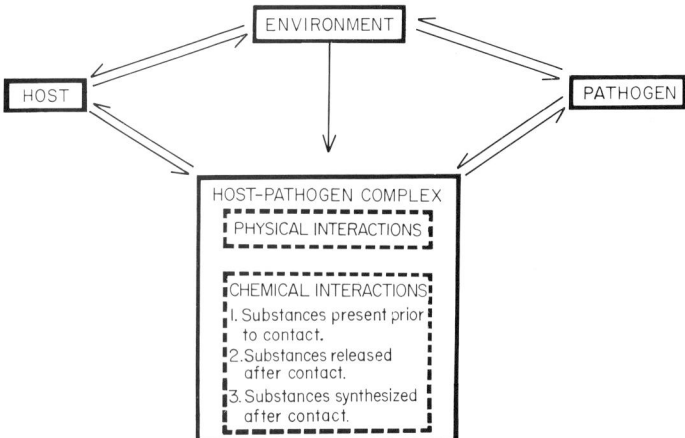

Figure 8.1 Host–pathogen interactions.

symptoms, especially in the case of biotrophic pathogens, which do not as a rule inflict much chemical damage.

This chapter is primarily concerned, however, with biochemical interactions taking place in the host–pathogen complex.

PROBLEMS IN IDENTIFYING THE NATURE OF BIOCHEMICAL INTERACTIONS

Living cells contain literally thousands of different types of organic molecules involved in the integrated reactions which make up metabolism. These reactions are mediated by enzymes and are ultimately controlled by the cell's genome. In diseases caused by bacteria and fungi, the host–pathogen complex comprises two different organisms, each with its own separate metabolism. The interactions between the two partners could therefore involve many different kinds of molecular reactions. Identification of the key interactions in biochemical terms is, not surprisingly, like looking for a needle in a haystack. Even in the case of virus infections, where the pathogen has a relatively simple molecular structure, the biochemistry of disease is far from fully understood.

According to our scheme shown in Fig. 8.1, three different categories of biochemical interaction are possible. The first, substances present prior to contact, is distinct inasmuch as no post-infectional changes in the metabolism of either the host or the pathogen are involved. The other categories both involve changes which occur after contact between host and pathogen.

Biochemistry of resistance

From a historical viewpoint, the early ideas concerning the differences between resistant and susceptible hosts envisaged that the critical factors were nutritional. According to this hypothesis the host is an inert substrate containing nutrients. Infection takes place if the host contains all the nutrients required by the pathogen. If not, the pathogen is unable to establish itself. Although this hypothesis has certain attractions, especially when considering nutritionally demanding biotrophic pathogens, there is little evidence to support it. Studies on *Venturia inaequalis* have shown that vitamin-requiring mutants are only virulent if inoculated into apple trees along with an exogenous supply of the appropriate vitamin. This observation is unlikely, however, to be relevant to the field situation, where the mutants would be unable to compete with non-vitamin-requiring wild-type strains. The successful axenic culture of rust fungi on relatively simple media has also cast doubt on the notion that nutritional factors determine the host range of biotrophic fungi.

More convincing experimental support was forthcoming, however, for an alternative hypothesis. Rather than explaining resistance in terms of the absence of essential nutrients, the host might contain toxic substances which prevent growth of the pathogen. As long ago as 1933, resistance of onions to *Colletotrichum circinans* was shown to be directly correlated with the presence in the pigmented outer scales of the phenolic compound, protocatechuic acid:

The discovery that a single compound, and a relatively simple one at that, is the basis of resistance to a plant pathogen provoked a search for similar chemical resistance factors in other plants. Few additional examples have been found. For instance, resistance of potato tubers to *Streptomyces scabies* appears to be correlated with high concentrations of another phenolic compound, chlorogenic acid.

The idea that preformed toxic compounds determine resistance falls within the first category of biochemical interactions in Fig. 8.1. Nutritional factors also belong here, although resistance in this case is determined by their absence rather than by their presence.

This review of some of the early ideas concerning the biochemistry of disease resistance leads one to the conclusion that the important interactions, in most cases, fall within the final two categories on our diagram (Fig. 8.1). Both of these categories involve the appearance of novel compounds in the host–pathogen complex after the two partners have come together. The implication is that the metabolism of the host, or the pathogen, or both, is altered by the presence of the other partner, and that these changes in turn control the outcome of the interaction.

At first sight the distinction between the final two categories, viz. substances released and substances synthesized, might appear academic.

138

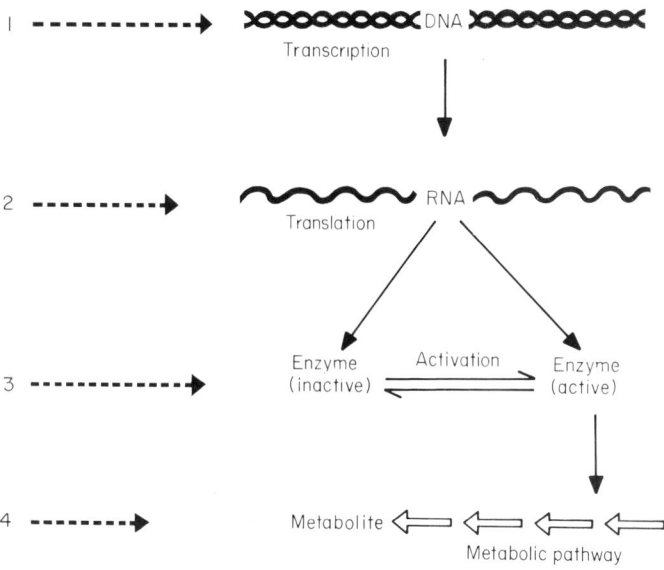

Figure 8.2 Scheme for genetic control of metabolism showing possible levels of interaction.

However, the former concerns substances released into the host–pathogen complex, perhaps as a result of alterations in membrane permeability and cellular compartmentation, while the latter implies changes in the activity of specific host or pathogen genes. Consideration of the accepted scheme for the regulation of cellular metabolism should clarify this distinction (Fig. 8.2). Genetic information contained in the DNA genome is expressed via RNA and protein synthesis, and ultimately determines the various metabolic products of anabolic or catabolic pathways. The diagram indicates a number of points at which metabolism may be altered.

Alterations in the pattern of genetic activity could occur either in the regulation of transcription itself, in other words at the level of DNA (1) or alternatively in the translation of genetic messengers on the ribosome (2). Previously inactive enzymes may be activated and alter the rate or direction of various metabolic pathways (3) or new compounds may also be released into the host cell by the pathogen (4). Neither of the latter interactions involves changes in the activity of genes. In practice, it may be very difficult to establish whether the primary interactions are at the level of the gene. There are, however, some obvious exceptions to this statement. Virus infection involves the introduction of a genetic messenger, usually RNA, into the host cell. Similarly there is now good evidence that infection by the crown gall bacterium involves the incorporation of bacterial DNA into the host cell (see below).

As was pointed out in Chapter 3, host resistance and pathogen virulence are properties controlled by one or a number of genes. This is merely stating the obvious as the characteristics of all organisms are genetically determined, although the expression of individual genes may be modified by the environment. It would be surprising if an event as drastic as the entry of a foreign organism had no effect on the host genome. However, the implications of the gene-for-gene concept (see Fig. 3.2) go further than this. If for each gene controlling host resistance there is a corresponding gene determining the degree of virulence of the pathogen, then the interaction between these genes or their products is highly specific. It has been postulated that the products of a pathogen gene for virulence might regulate the activity of a host gene for resistance, and vice versa. The problem in proving this hypothesis is that although in many cases we know the number of genes controlling resistance or virulence their biochemical functions have not yet been identified. Presumably the genes produce proteins, but whether these function as enzymes or interact as receptor molecules with products from the other partner is not known. There is the further possibility that genetic messengers produced by these genes may pass from one partner to the other, acting either as activators or repressors, or otherwise redirecting the metabolism of the recipient cell. Several schemes along these lines have been suggested but, in the absence of experimental evidence, they remain highly speculative.

Much of the preceding discussion is probably only relevant to diseases involving biotrophic pathogens, where there is a high degree of host specificity and where the host–pathogen interface involves two living cells. Necrotrophic pathogens kill host cells relatively quickly through the action of toxins or hydrolytic enzymes. It is unlikely therefore, that subtle interactions involving informational macromolecules can occur. This does not, however, preclude the possibility that molecular interactions also control specificity in diseases caused by these pathogens.

HIGH-MOLECULAR-WEIGHT COMPOUNDS IN HOST–PATHOGEN INTERACTION

Three major classes of high-molecular-weight compounds are found in living cells—nucleic acids, proteins and polysaccharides. Because of their key position in the direction and regulation of metabolism it seems likely that many of the biochemical changes in infected tissues can be traced to changes in the nucleic acids and proteins. This is especially so in biotrophic relationships where a redirection of host metabolism occurs. Polysaccharides are principally of importance as storage compounds and as components of plant cell walls. For this reason, interest in these compounds has mainly concerned necrotrophic pathogens, which produce extracellular polysaccharases capable of degrading plant polymers. One should also note that polysaccharide components of fungal cell walls and the cell envelope of plant pathogenic bacteria have now been implicated in the induction of host defence mechanisms (see Chapter 9).

NUCLEIC ACIDS

The acceleration of metabolism in diseased tissues is usually accompanied by an increased synthesis of RNA, and consequently of protein as well. Thus, cells penetrated by fungal haustoria or from the periphery of disease lesions often contain more polyribosomes than healthy cells, suggesting that protein synthesis is enhanced. This conclusion is supported by observations on the nucleoli of infected cells, which typically are swollen indicating an accumulation of RNA. If one measures the rate of incorporation of radioactive phosphorus into the RNA fraction of wheat leaves infected by the stem rust fungus, the rate of RNA synthesis is almost three times that found in healthy leaves (Fig. 8.3). However, it should be noted that this stimulation

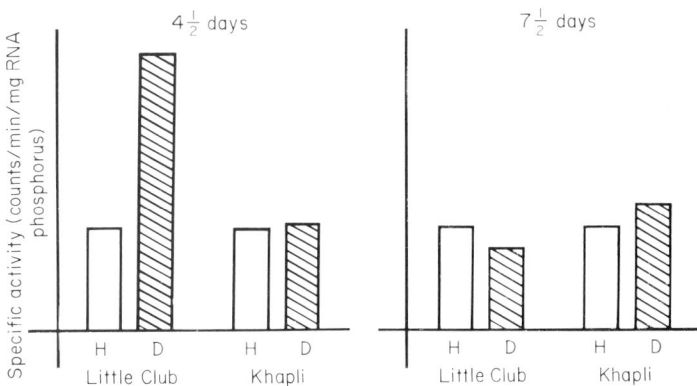

Figure 8.3 Amount of ^{32}P incorporated into RNA of wheat leaves cv Little Club (susceptible) and cv Khapli (resistant) inoculated with *Puccinia graminis*. H = healthy, D = diseased leaves. (Data from Rohringer & Heitefuss, 1961.)

of RNA synthesis is restricted to early stages of infection; after longer periods, the rate of incorporation is actually lower than that in healthy leaves. Furthermore, in resistant leaves RNA synthesis is apparently unchanged. This suggests that the higher levels of RNA synthesis in the infected leaves are only characteristic of the compatible host–pathogen combination at a stage when the fungus is beginning to sporulate. The additional nucleic acid synthesis would be entirely due to synthesis by the pathogen.

One omission in these data should be apparent. The resistant reaction would be expected to be complete by four days, in which case any changes correlated with this response would be overlooked. In fact, inoculation of cereal leaves with an avirulent race of a rust fungus leads to an early increase in RNA synthesis. Treatment with inhibitors of RNA synthesis has been shown to depress resistance to crown rust of oats. Further support for the idea that induction of resistance involves activation of host genes has come from recent work on the accumulation of inhibitory compounds known as phytoalexins; production of at least some of these compounds is accompanied by *de novo* synthesis of messenger RNA and protein (see later in this chapter).

Thus, there is good evidence that infection by pathogens leads to changes in the activity of the host genome. The mechanism involved in the 'switching on' or 'switching off' of genes in eukaryotic cells is still not clear; some authors envisage a role for the class of nuclear proteins known as histones. In this context it may be significant that changes in the histone fraction of host cells have been detected in several host–pathogen combinations, including diseases caused by rusts, powdery mildews, and club root.

In view of their function as informational macromolecules, it is hardly surprising that nucleic acids should have been postulated as the primary interactants in a gene-for-gene system. Some research has suggested that RNA extracted from wheat leaves undergoing a hypersensitive response to infection by the stem rust fungus can induce a necrotic reaction in similar leaves infected with a compatible race of the pathogen. If verified, this is a significant discovery as the active RNA showed the same specificity as the host–pathogen system itself. Further work has suggested that the RNA involved may be the product of the pathogen avirulence gene which specifically interacts with the corresponding host gene for resistance. However, as we saw in Chapter 7, necrosis may be an unreliable indicator of resistance, and doubts remain over the interpretation of these experiments.

Nucleic acids in gall-forming diseases

A number of plant pathogens interfere with cell growth and division, and give rise to malformations in the host. It seems reasonable to suppose that these symptoms are accompanied by some derangement of the genetic machinery of the host. The galls formed during infection of maize by *Ustilago maydis* (see Fig. 6.2) result from hyperplasia of host cells; hyperplastic cells from within the gall contain swollen nuclei which have an increased DNA content. Similar changes are also evident in hypertrophied cells from club root galls (see Fig. 2.2). In this case, nucleolar volumes may increase 30-fold, and the DNA content 16-fold. Within two hours of the pathogen entering root-hair cells there is an increase in the level of root-hair RNA. The massive increases in DNA content are, however, restricted to cells within the galls which are formed as a result of secondary infections of the root cortex.

Bacterial pathogens can also induce growth deformities, the best-known example being *Agrobacterium tumefaciens* which causes crown galls in many plants. Crown gall disease is of particular interest as, following the initial infection through a wound, secondary galls are formed which do not contain the pathogen. These tumours are, therefore, autonomous and bear some resemblance to animal cancers. In comparison with healthy cells, tumour cells exhibit differences in their pattern of nucleic acid synthesis. However, the major debate concerns the identity of the factor which transforms host cells into tumour cells. It was originally postulated that some component of the bacterium, the 'tumour-inducing principle', enters the host cell and somehow alters the regulation of the host genome. The most likely candidate for this role was a nucleic acid.

The past decade has seen spectacular advances in our understanding of tumour induction in the crown gall disease. First it was demonstrated that virulent strains of *Agrobacterium* all contain a large plasmid, known as the tumour-inducing or Ti plasmid. As well as carrying the genes for virulence, the Ti plasmid also codes for some unusual amino acids, the opines, which can be detected in tumour tissues. Ingenious genetic analyses have shown that a small part of the plasmid is transferred to the host cell, where it is integrated into host DNA in the nucleus, transcribed and replicated. It is not yet known if transcription of plasmid DNA is a prerequisite for transformation of the host cell; should integration into the host genome occur at certain crucial positions it is conceivable that this alone might be sufficient to disrupt the control of cell division. Studies on transformed cells grown in tissue culture have shown that the plasmid DNA is stable over many generations, and there have even been some indications that it will pass through meiosis.

In essence, the crown gall bacterium is a naturally occurring 'genetic engineer'. It is able to transform host cells and programme them to produce unusual amino acids, which are a food source for the pathogen. This property is of great interest to biologists seeking novel ways of modifying the genetic content of plant cells (see Chapter 10). Intriguingly, it also bears similarities to the induction of animal cancers by oncogenic viruses, where insertion of foreign DNA into the host cell leads to malignant transformation.

Nucleic acids in virus infection

The nucleic acid metabolism of virus-infected plant cells represents a special case in that the infective part of the virus is itself a nucleic acid. Characteristically, there is an increase in the nucleic acid content of virus-infected cells, but it should be borne in mind that this increase could represent changes in the amount of several components, including host DNA and RNA, as well as viral nucleic acid. In tobacco leaves infected by TMV, there is an increase in RNA synthesis within two hours of inoculation. Subsequently, however, there is a severe inhibition of cellular RNA synthesis, accompanied by the breakdown of some types of host RNA, such as chloroplast ribosomal RNA. The degradation of host RNA, coupled with an inhibition of its synthesis, presumably ensures that there is an adequate pool of nucleic acid precursors available for virus replication.

Plant viruses have evolved several strategies to ensure their successful replication within host cells. Although the sequence of molecular events varies from one class of virus to another and different intracellular sites of replication, such as nuclei, plastids or vesicles, may be involved, the end result is similar. The biosynthetic machinery of the host cell is subverted and redirected into the manufacture of new virus particles.

As we saw in Chapter 4, viroids are small infectious RNA molecules lacking any coat protein. Although the mode of replication of viroids remains obscure, it seems unlikely that viroid RNA has a messenger function. Instead, after migrating to the nucleus, the viroid may interact with the host genome in some regulatory capacity. Due to the minimal genetic information present in viroid RNA, replication must be highly host dependent.

PROTEINS

The genetic information contained in nucleic acids is expressed in the cell via the synthesis of proteins. Many proteins function as enzymes in the metabolic pathways which synthesize or break down cellular materials.

In keeping with the general pattern of enhanced metabolic activity in infected plants, the total nitrogen and protein content of the host–pathogen complex is usually higher than that found in uninfected parts of the host. For example, in wheat leaves infected by *Puccinia graminis* there is a striking increase in the nitrogen content at infection sites, part of which is due to a synthesis of new protein. In rusted bean leaves the rate of incorporation of radioactively labelled amino acids into disease lesions is twice that occurring in non-infected regions of the leaf. Studies on the fate of these amino acids have shown that they are mainly incorporated into the fungus. Much of the increased synthesis of protein can therefore be attributed to the pathogen, and it appears that, as well as accumulating host sugars, biotrophic pathogens are able to divert amino acids to their own ends.

While the compatible host–pathogen combination is characterized by an increased synthesis of cellular materials including proteins, the situation with resistant hosts is much less clear. An increase in protein synthesis is in some cases the first detectable expression of the resistant reaction, for instance in flax inoculated with incompatible races of the rust *Melampsora lini*. In contrast, no obvious changes in the soluble protein content of wheat leaves have been detected during the resistance response to leaf or stem rust. Similar negative results have been obtained with oats inoculated with crown rust. This latter result is perplexing as we have already seen that there is a pronounced increase in RNA synthesis which is not therefore correlated with changes in the amount of protein present. Instead this enhanced RNA synthesis may be linked to qualitative changes in proteins. According to this explanation, resistance is not mediated by a large increase in protein synthesis but rather by the synthesis of a few specific proteins by the host.

The effects of virus infection on the host's protein metabolism vary according to the virus concerned and the severity of the infection. In tobacco infected by TMV, at least one-third of the total nitrogen may eventually be present in virus particles. Total nitrogen is increased during infection, but this is coupled with a net breakdown of host protein. Most viruses do not, however, multiply to this extent within the host and only an insignificant portion of the total nitrogen present may be bound up in viral protein. In these cases, hard overall effects of infection are to evaluate.

Measurement of gross changes in the total nitrogen or protein content of infected plants does not provide any information on alterations in the type of protein present. The development of more sensitive techniques for protein analysis, such as electrophoresis, column chromatography and immunological methods, has meant that we are now able to detect changes in specific types of protein. It is clear that information on changes in the amount of particular enzymes can tell us much more about the nature of pathogenesis and disease resistance than measurement of overall protein concentration.

It has been known for some time that new types of protein occur in and around disease lesions. Using a combination of electrophoresis and immunochemistry, early workers were able to show that new protein antigens were present in cabbage seedlings infected by *Fusarium oxysporum* f. sp. *conglutinans*, and in sweet potatoes infected by *Ceratocystis fimbriata*. Similar antigens could be detected in uninfected cells adjacent to invaded tissues, suggesting that the new proteins were being synthesized by the host. The important conclusion to be drawn from this work was that resistance might be correlated with changes in the protein metabolism of the host.

Enzymes

If one prepares protein extracts from infected plant tissues and assays the activity of a number of enzymes, one can invariably detect changes in some or all of them when compared with healthy tissues. Furthermore, by subjecting the extracts to electrophoresis or column chromatography, one can often identify different molecular forms (or isoenzymes) present in diseased plants. For instance, in barley leaves infected with *Erysiphe graminis*, 11 out of 14 enzymes studied were found to be altered during infection. Most of these changes represented increases in the activity of particular isoenzymes. Similar results have been obtained with diseases caused by bacteria and viruses, the activity of several enzymes being stimulated in cells around disease lesions. These changes can be thought of as biochemical symptoms of disease, but little purpose would be served by attempting to list them all. Instead we should try to identify those enzymes which seem to play a prominent role in disease, in relation either to symptom development or to host resistance responses.

A number of enzymes have been the subject of special attention, either because their activity is conspicuously altered following infection or because changes in these enzymes seem to be a universal feature of diseases caused by a wide variety of pathogens. Such enzymes include several in the pentose phosphate pathway (such as glucose-6-phosphate dehydrogenase), oxidases (such as polyphenol oxidase and peroxidase) and a key enzyme in phenolic biosynthesis (phenylalanine ammonia lyase or PAL). In addition, some hydrolases, especially ribonuclease, exhibit considerably increased activity in infected tissues. The activity of all these enzymes is also increased in injured tissues, suggesting that their induction and/or activation is part of a non-specific stress response by the plant.

If, as was suggested earlier, the higher respiratory rate of infected tissues involves an enhanced participation by the pentose phosphate pathway, then commensurate increases in the activity of enzymes involved in this pathway are predictable. What is of greater interest is that pentose phosphate pathway intermediates, such as erythrose phosphate, provide the starting point for the major pathway for biosynthesis of phenolic compounds, viz. the shikimic acid pathway (Fig. 8.4). It would be misleading, however, to assume that pentose pathway enzymes are the only respiratory enzymes affected during infection. For example, activity of malate dehydrogenase,

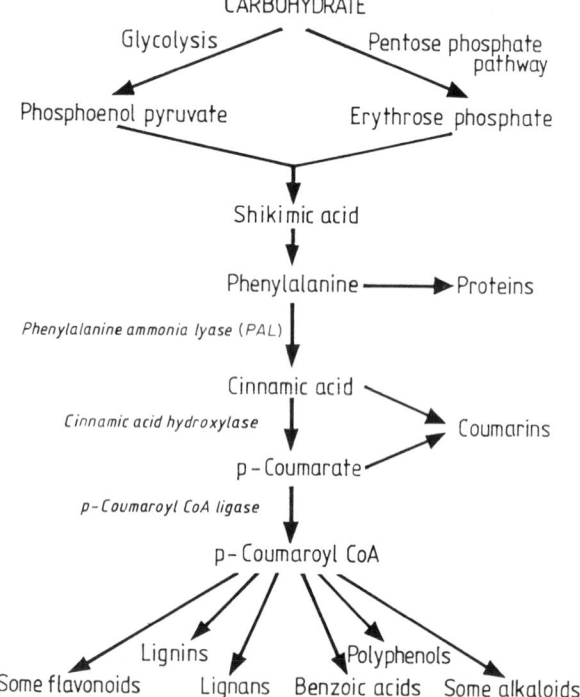

Figure 8.4 Shikimic acid pathway and the biosynthesis of phenolic compounds.

which is a TCA-cycle enzyme, can also be stimulated. In peas infected by *Fusarium*, activity is increased by almost 300%, together with the appearance of a new molecular form of this enzyme which is unique to the host–pathogen complex.

Enzymes involved in phenol metabolism

A wide variety of phenolic compounds accumulate in infected plants, and

146

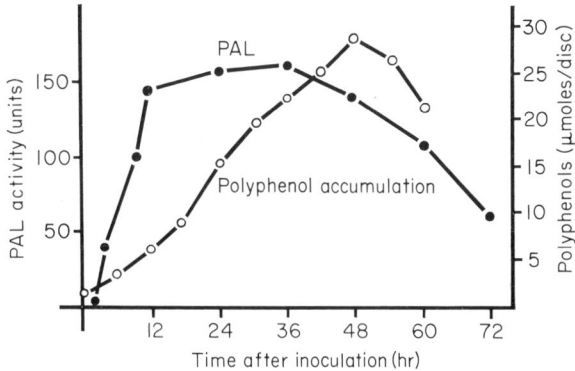

Figure 8.5 Activity of PAL and polyphenol accumulation in discs of sweet potato tissue following inoculation with *Ceratocystis fimbriata* (data from Minamikawa & Uritani, 1964).

many of them inhibit the growth of pathogens. For this reason, enzymes involved in the biosynthesis of phenols are of special interest. A key step in the shikimic acid pathway is the deamination of phenylalanine to cinnamic acid. This is a branch point at which material is diverted from protein synthesis to phenylpropanoid metabolism (Fig. 8.4). The enzyme involved in the reaction is PAL and its activity has been shown to increase in response to a number of stimuli, including light and mechanical injury as well as infection by fungi, bacteria and virus strains which induce local lesions. Within 24 hours of infection by *Ceratocystis fimbriata*, PAL activity in sweet potato tissue rises to a peak, and this increase is followed by a rise in the concentration of polyphenols (Fig. 8.5). A similar time-course of events occurs if the tissues are sliced, rather than infected by the fungus. Because an increase in PAL activity seems to be a non-specific stress response, the relationship of this enzyme to resistance is hard to evaluate. However, in potato tubers infected by blight, the increase in PAL and the associated build-up of chlorogenic acid and lignin take place more rapidly in cultivars exhibiting a hypersensitive reaction. It has also been shown that the accumulation of the phytoalexin phaseollin (see p. 159) in French-bean cells is accompanied by a transient increase in PAL activity, and that this increase is due to a *de novo* synthesis of the enzyme.

While emphasis has been placed on PAL, recent evidence suggests that the activities of two related enzymes which catalyse subsequent steps in the shikimic acid pathway (cinnamic acid hydroxylase and p-coumaroyl CoA ligase; Fig. 8.4) also increase in response to various injurious agents. This coordinated stimulation of several enzymes indicates that the whole pathway is operating at a higher level in diseased tissues.

A common indication of pathological metabolism is some discolouration of the affected tissues. In certain cases this may even be a valuable diagnostic symptom, for instance the darkening of xylem tissue in plants infected by vascular wilt pathogens (Fig. 8.6). Although the biochemistry of the reaction is complex, the enzyme polyphenol oxidase, which converts polyphenolic compounds to quinones, is definitely involved. The rate of oxida-

147

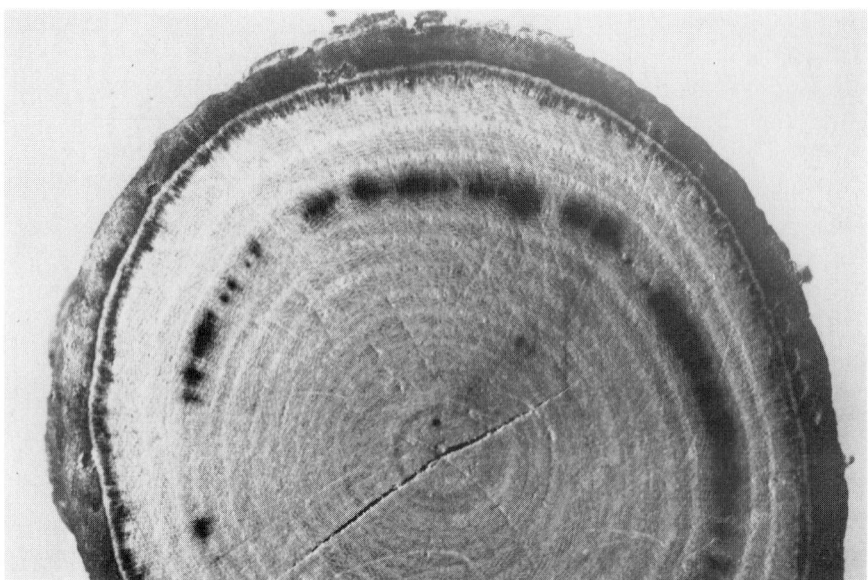

Figure 8.6 Cross-section of an elm branch showing dark spots in two annual rings. The tree has suffered two attacks of Dutch elm disease and the spots indicate reactions in the xylem caused by the pathogen (see also Fig. 7.13). (Photograph by courtesy of the Forestry Commission.)

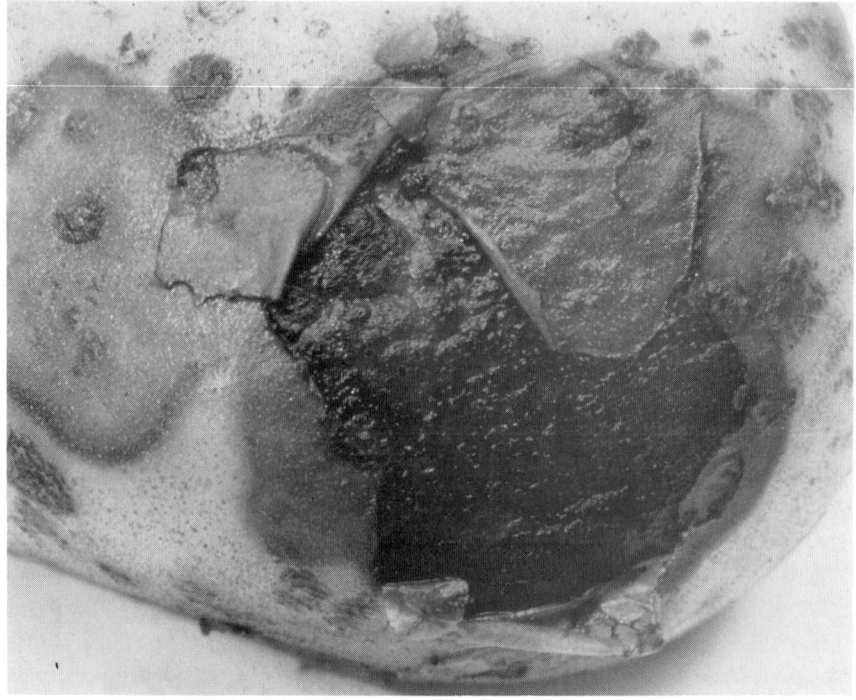

Figure 8.7 Soft-rot lesion in a potato tuber caused by the bacterium *Erwinia carotovora*.

tion of polyphenols is enhanced in tissues adjacent to disease lesions, and this may create an inhibitory zone which is an effective barrier to further spread of the pathogen. Localization of *Erwinia carotovora* in potato tubers is accompanied by the development of a conspicuous black margin around the invaded tissues (Fig. 8.7). Polyphenol oxidase has also been implicated in the local lesion reaction to viruses, as activity of this enzyme increases during necrosis. A similar pattern is seen with the enzyme peroxidase, activity in this case being almost ten times that in healthy leaves in the zone adjacent to the local lesion (Fig. 8.8).

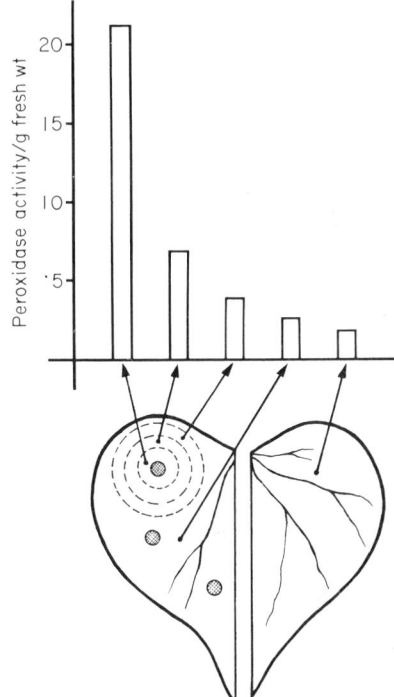

Figure 8.8 Peroxidase activity in successive 1-mm zones around local lesions in leaves of *Nicotiana tabacum* var. *xanthi* 10 days after inoculation with TMV. Values for tissues between lesions and for tissue from uninfected leaves are also shown. (Data from Weststeijn, 1976.)

The role of peroxidase in disease has been the subject of much research, as increased activity seems to be an almost universal feature of tissues infected by fungi, bacteria and viruses. Although stimulation of peroxidase activity is once again non-specific, there is persuasive evidence for a correlation between high peroxidase activity and resistance. A more rapid and marked increase is found in resistant hosts, and the phenomenon of acquired immunity (see Chapter 9) also seems to be linked to increases in peroxidase activity. Definite conclusions are hampered by the lack of information on the role played by peroxidase in plant cells. One possibility is that peroxidase plays a part in the lignification of host cell walls, but conclusive evidence for this is lacking. However, changes in enzymes involved in the biosynthesis and oxidation of phenolic compounds undoubtedly contribute to the creation of a cellular environment which is inhibitory to invading micro-organisms.

Hydrolases

Another group of enzymes which is of great importance in plant disease comprises the hydrolases which break down complex substances into simpler compounds. Not surprisingly, these enzymes are often implicated in necrotrophic diseases, where the digestion of host tissues is a prominent feature of pathogenesis. However, hydrolases may also be of significance in biotrophic associations. For instance, invertase activity is increased in tissues surrounding rust pustules, and this enzyme is believed to play a part in the uptake of soluble sugars by the pathogen. Similarly, the level of amylase, which degrades starch to maltose, increases in response to infection by a wide variety of pathogens. Another enzyme which may be dramatically increased in infected tissues is ribonuclease. In virus-infected plants, this enzyme may play an important role in the processing of viral or host RNA, including degradation of the latter to furnish nucleotides for the synthesis of new viral nucleic acid. Increases in its level of activity are also seen in diseases caused by bacteria and fungi. Figure 8.9 shows that two days after

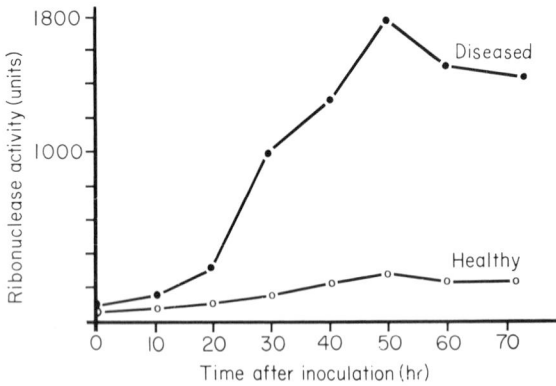

Figure 8.9 Ribonuclease activity in healthy potato leaves and leaves affected by *Phytophthora infestans* (data from Pitt, 1976).

inoculation with potato blight the ribonuclease activity of potato leaves reaches a peak. It is not clear whether this large increase coincides with an increase in the pool of nucleotides available to the fungus. Rather, analysis of ribonuclease in blighted potato leaves highlights the complexity of what would at first sight appear to be a relatively simple phenomenon. Several different molecular forms of the enzyme seem to be involved, some of which are similar to host enzymes while others appear to originate from the fungus. In addition, one should bear in mind the fact that increases in overall activity may be of less significance than changes in the intracellular distribution of an enzyme.

In healthy cells, there is a balance between the synthesis of new materials and the degradation of components which are no longer required. Thus, there is a continual turnover of proteins, nucleic acids and other materials, with the essential building blocks being recycled. This breakdown of obsolete macromolecules is carried out by specific digestive enzymes, such as ribonuclease, and proteases. Indiscriminate action by these enzymes would have disastrous consequences for the cell, so they are usually compartmentalized in vacuoles or lysosomes. During disease, however, this balance may be upset, with the result that hydrolytic enzymes are released into the cell. In the example above, potatoes affected by *Phytophthora infestans*, leaf necrosis is accompanied by a release of lysosomal enzymes into the soluble phase of the cell cytoplasm. A similar sequence of events is seen in potato tubers infected by a number of soft-rot pathogens. Thus it appears that the host cells contribute to their own fate by liberating previously latent digestive enzymes which presumably act in much the same way as extracellular enzymes produced by the pathogen. The self-same mechanism might, however, work to the host's advantage in a resistance reaction, such as the hypersensitive response, which involves very rapid cellular necrosis. Lysosomal breakdown has, in fact, been suggested as a basis for hypersensitive cell death, but it is difficult to establish whether the release of hydrolytic enzymes actually triggers the process or is merely a consequence of degenerative changes set in motion by some other lethal event.

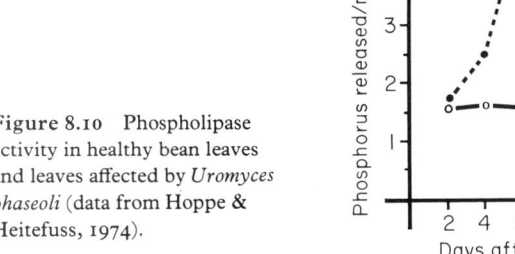

Figure 8.10 Phospholipase activity in healthy bean leaves and leaves affected by *Uromyces phaseoli* (data from Hoppe & Heitefuss, 1974).

The release of enzymes from lysosomes is another example of a change in cellular membrane systems following infection. As we discussed in the last chapter, many aspects of disease physiology may eventually be explained in terms of alterations in the properties of membranes. Among the many agents capable of modifying or destroying cell membranes are enzymes such as phospholipase. Changes in phospholipase activity have been recorded in infected plants, such as bean leaves infected by *Uromyces phaseoli* (Fig. 8.10). Phospholipase also seems to be involved in a number of necrotrophic diseases, although here there is good evidence that the enzyme is a product of the pathogen rather than the host. In fact, this is a convenient point at which to consider the contribution of the pathogen to the enzymology of the host–pathogen complex.

Enzymes produced by the pathogen

Micro-organisms, with the obvious exception of the viruses, are noted for their ability to produce extracellular enzymes, often in large amounts. Pathogenic species are no exception to this, and many produce enzymes which assist in the colonization of the host. While it is often difficult to assess the relative contributions of the host and the pathogen to the changes observed in diseased plants, in some cases it is clear that the principal symptoms are due to the action of enzymes secreted by the pathogen. The best-known examples are the diseases of plant storage tissues commonly described as soft-rots.

Almost one hundred years ago, De Bary showed that extracts of rotted plant tissue can macerate firm, healthy tissues. This phenomenon was further investigated during the early part of this century by William Brown at Imperial College who, in a series of classic papers, showed that the maceration of host tissues was due to the action of cell-separating enzymes produced by the pathogen. These enzymes degrade the pectic substances in the middle lamella between cells, thereby facilitating the colonization of host tissues. The ability to produce pectolytic enzymes is widely distributed amongst fungi and bacteria and is characteristic of necrotrophic pathogens such as *Botrytis*, *Sclerotinia* and *Erwinia*.

Brown recognized that the soft-rot syndrome involved two processes. Host cells within the lesion were separated through the action of enzymes, and then the cells died. Brown proposed two alternative theories to explain these processes.

1 Host cells are separated and killed by the same substance, i.e. the macerating factor and the lethal factor are identical.

2 Host cells are separated by the action of the macerating factor and subsequently killed by a different lethal factor, for instance a toxin of some kind.

In his experiments Brown was unable to separate macerating activity from lethal activity, a result which favoured the first hypothesis. However, in spite of a considerable amount of further research, there is still debate on this problem.

Figure 8.11 shows the results of an experiment similar to those which originally highlighted the problem. Discs of potato tuber tissue were treated with an extract of another tuber which had been rotted by *Erwinia carotovora*. As can be seen, this extract was very active in killing potato cells. At the same time, tuber discs were also treated with filtrates from cultures of the bacterium grown either on a potato medium or on the same medium supplemented with pectin. The pectin medium filtrate was almost as toxic to cells as the original rot extract, while the other filtrate had virtually no effect. As the bacterium produces much greater amounts of pectolytic enzymes on the pectin medium this result suggests that the macerating enzymes are also responsible, directly or indirectly, for cell death. The problem with this experiment, like many others investigating host cell death, is that the extract and filtrates are crude mixtures of enzymes and other potentially

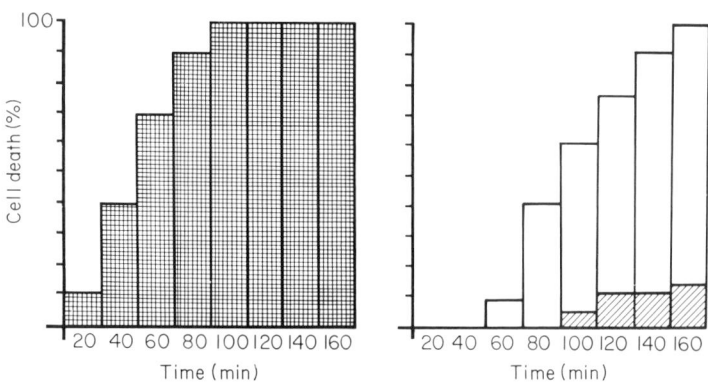

Figure 8.11   Lethal activity of *Erwinia* rot extract (▦) and culture filtrates from potato medium (▨) and potato medium supplemented with pectin (□).

active components, and the result is, therefore, inconclusive. Much more critical work, in which the different components are isolated and purified, is needed to resolve the problem. In recent years considerable progress has been made towards this end, but the situation remains complex, largely because soft-rot pathogens produce not one but a whole series of wall-degrading enzymes, each with a slightly different mode of action. For instance, pectin methyl esterases remove the methyl groups of pectin to yield pectic acid, which is then more susceptible to polygalacturonases which actually cleave the polymer into galacturonic acid. Synthesis of these enzymes may be induced or repressed by catabolites in a highly specific manner, so that critical attention must be paid to the culture media used. In addition to the pectolytic enzymes there are also enzymes which attack other wall polymers, such as cellulases, hemicellulases and ligninases. These latter types are generally considered to be important in diseases involving wood decay, such as heart rots of trees. In combination these enzymes can degrade all the polysaccharides present in higher plant cell walls.

To return to the problem of the lethal factor, it is now known with reasonable certainty that purified pectolytic enzymes can, in isolation, kill host cells as well as macerating the tissues. One example is shown in Fig. 8.12 where the activity of a single enzyme from *Erwinia*, isolated by electrophoresis, is shown to correspond with lethal activity towards potato cells. The way in which the enzyme actually kills host cells is, however, still open to debate. Recent evidence favours the hypothesis that cell walls in plant tissues treated with pectic enzymes lose their ability to support the plasma membrane, particularly under osmotic stress. Direct effects of reaction products of the enzyme on the cells do not appear to be responsible for cell death.

We have devoted so much space to pectic enzymes because they have been the subject of much research and controversy for almost a century. It should be emphasized, however, that although these enzymes are of great significance in soft-rot diseases and have been implicated in vascular wilt

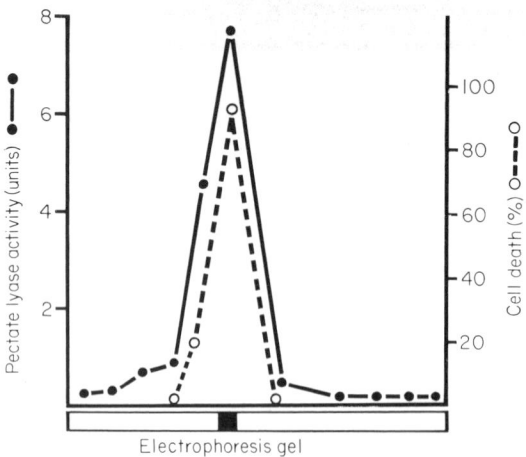

Figure 8.12 Separation of a pectolytic enzyme (endopectate lyase) from *Erwinia* by acrylamide gel electrophoresis. The enzyme has migrated in the gel as a single band. Note that high enzyme activity (●) coincides with greatest lethal activity (○) towards potato cells. (Data from Basham & Bateman, 1975.)

syndromes, many pathogens do not macerate host tissues and have negligible effects on pectic substances. In these diseases, other enzymes, or alternatively low-molecular-weight compounds such as toxins, may be more important. Even in certain soft-rot diseases there is reason to believe that enzymes active towards other cellular substrates, such as phospholipases and proteases, also play a part in pathogenesis. Finally it should be remembered that the enzymic degradation of host tissues by the pathogen is not usually a feature of biotrophic infections.

We should conclude this discussion on enzymes produced by the pathogen by asking to what extent secretion of these enzymes can be correlated with virulence. Generally speaking there is little evidence to suggest that the successful pathogen is the one which produces most enzyme. Instead, the ability of certain cell wall proteins in the host to inhibit pectolytic enzymes may contribute to the general level of host resistance to soft-rot pathogens (see Chapter 9).

LOW-MOLECULAR-WEIGHT COMPOUNDS IN HOST–PATHOGEN INTERACTION

Low-molecular-weight compounds of significance in host–pathogen interactions can conveniently be discussed in the section under three headings: toxins, which are produced by the pathogen; phytoalexins, which are produced by the host; and growth regulators, which are produced by both partners.

Toxins

The idea that pathogenesis might be due to the production of poisons by the pathogen is by no means new, but only in recent years has it been put on a firm scientific basis. Many pathogens growing *in vitro* secrete substances which, when introduced into the host plant, reproduce some or all of the symptoms associated with infection by that pathogen. Because these substances are capable of disrupting metabolism they are described as TOXINS. In theory the term can refer to any pathogen product which is harmful to the host, including the hydrolytic enzymes we discussed in the previous section. In practice it is usually restricted to low-molecular-weight compounds which do not attack the structural integrity of plant tissues but instead affect metabolism in some other, more subtle fashion. A useful working definition is 'a metabolite of pathogen origin which is involved in plant disease'. Two important properties of toxins are (1) that they are active in very low concentrations, and (2) that they are mobile within the plant, and may, therefore, act at a distance from the actual site of infection.

Experimental proof that a toxin is involved in a particular disease is tricky for a number of reasons. The demonstration that a compound produced in culture can cause disease symptoms is not in itself conclusive evidence because there is no guarantee that the same compound is produced *in vivo*. To overcome this problem a set of rules, somewhat akin to Koch's postulates, have been proposed to confirm the involvement of a toxin in a disease syndrome. In essence these rules insist that the suspected toxin must be isolated from the diseased host, purified, and re-introduced with subsequent development of the same symptoms. Needless to say, these rules are of limited use in practice because a toxin may only be present in tiny amounts or may be so unstable that it breaks down during extraction. However, the importance of toxins in a number of plant diseases is now beyond doubt, and every year further compounds are added to the list.

Toxins known to play a causal role in disease have been termed PATHOTOXINS. Two main categories of pathotoxin are now recognized (Table 8.1), host-specific (selective) and non-specific (non-selective).

Table 8.1 Some toxins involved in plant disease.

	Toxin	Pathogen	Host
1. Host-specific (selective)	Victorin	*Helminthosporium victoriae*	Oats
	T toxin	*Helminthosporium maydis* Race T	Maize
	Helminthosporoside	*Helminthosporium sacchari*	Sugarcane
	PC toxin	*Periconia circinata*	Sorghum
	Phytoalternarin	*Alternaria kikuchiana*	Japanese pear
2. Non-specific (non-selective)	Fusicoccin	*Fusicoccum amygdali*	Almond
	Tentoxin	*Alternaria alternata*	Cotton and others
	Ophiobolin	*Helminthosporium oryzae*	Rice
	Wildfire toxin (Tabtoxin)	*Pseudomonas tabaci*	Tobacco
	Phaseolotoxin	*Pseudomonas phaseolicola*	Bean

Host-specific toxins

In 1946, oat crops in the USA were affected by a seedling blight caused by *Helminthosporium victoriae*. The fungus was especially virulent on one cultivar known as Victoria. Although the pathogen itself was typically localized in the basal portion of infected plants, symptoms extended into the leaves, which often collapsed. Suspicions that a mobile toxin was responsible were strengthened when it was shown that fungal-culture filtrates caused the same symptoms. The compound involved was named victorin, and it was isolated and characterized as a peptide linked to a tricyclic amine. What was particularly interesting about this toxin was that resistant oat cultivars were not affected by it, while cultivars such as Victoria were sensitive to extremely low concentrations (Fig. 8.13). In other words, the toxin

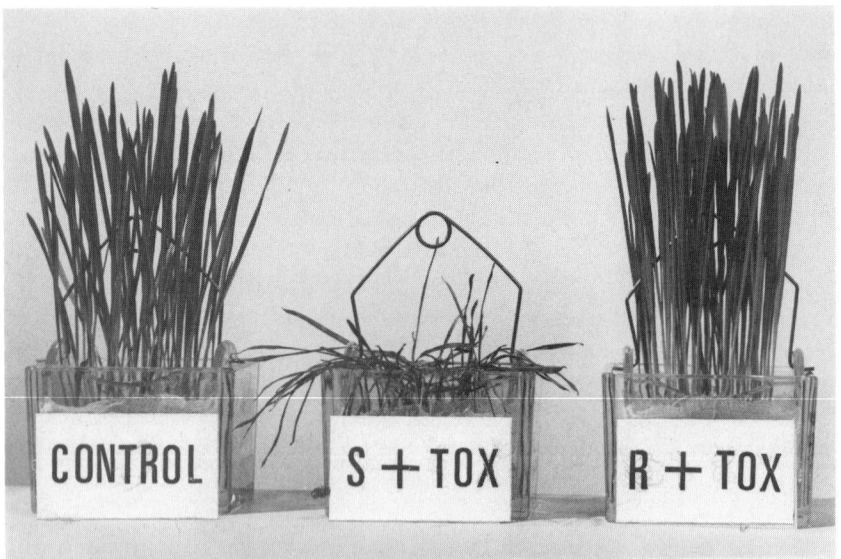

Figure 8.13 Effect of victorin on resistant (R) and susceptible (S) oat seedlings. Toxin was added to the nutrient solution where indicated, three days before the photograph was taken. (After Scheffer & Yoder, 1972.)

showed the same specificity as the pathogen itself. In addition, there was a direct correlation between toxin production and virulence; only toxin-producing strains of the fungus were pathogenic. All this evidence pointed to victorin as the sole determinant of the disease.

Victorin has widespread physiological effects in the host. It stimulates respiration, the increase being directly proportional to the concentration of toxin applied to the plant. Although the mechanism of its toxicity is not fully established, a major effect seems to be on cell permeability (Fig. 8.14). Damage to the cell plasma membrane has been observed in electron micrographs of victorin-treated cells. What has not yet been resolved is whether the plasma membrane is the primary site of action.

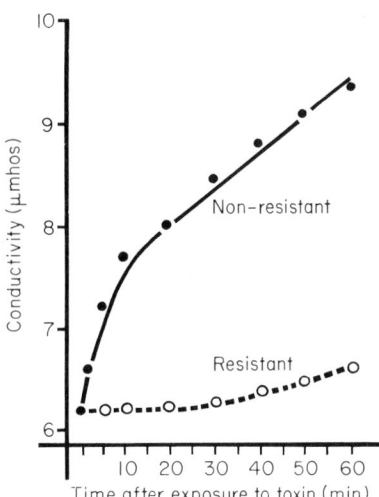

Figure 8.14 Effect of victorin on loss of electrolytes from resistant and non-resistant oat tissue (data from Samaddar & Scheffer, 1971).

The mode of action of a host-specific toxin has been analysed more thoroughly in the case of eyespot disease of sugar cane, caused by *Helminthosporium sacchari*. As the name implies, this pathogen gives rise to characteristic eye-shaped lesions, from which reddish-brown runners extend up the leaf. These runners do not contain the fungus and result from the translocation of a toxin, helminthosporoside. Like victorin, all aspects of pathogenesis may be ascribed to this single compound, which is suspected of being related to plant galactosides such as raffinose. In fact, if host leaves are pretreated with alpha-galactosides, they are protected against subsequent exposure to the toxin. This observation led Strobel to investigate the site of action of the toxin in host cells. By radioactively labelling the toxin he was able to trace its fate and show that it is specifically bound to a membrane fraction. In resistant cultivars, less binding of toxin was observed; bound toxin could be released from the membrane fraction by protease treatment, suggesting that the specific binding site was proteinaceous in nature. Strobel went on to isolate alpha-galactoside-binding proteins from the membranes of resistant and susceptible sugarcane plants and demonstrated minor differences in their amino acid composition. These differences, originally believed to involve as few as four amino acid residues, determine whether or not helminthosporoside is bound. The harmful effects on the host cell appear to be due to a malfunction in the regulation of ion transport across the plasma membrane when toxin is bound.

A molecular model of pathogenesis in eyespot disease, based on these findings, has now been proposed. Specific binding of toxin to a membrane protein in susceptible plants disrupts the activity of a neighbouring ATPase enzyme which controls uptake of potassium ions. According to this model a single molecular event, namely recognition of a low-molecular-weight toxin by a protein located in the plasma membrane, is sufficient to set in motion the whole disease process.

If verified, this work represents a landmark in our understanding of host–pathogen interaction. The model provides a specific determinant of pathogenicity in the fungus, and an equally specific mechanism for susceptibility in the host. However, doubts have been expressed about the kinetics of toxin binding in the original experiments and certain paradoxes remain. For instance, alpha-galactoside-binding proteins from a diversity of non-host plants also bind toxin, yet these plants are resistant to the disease.

While most data suggest that the receptor sites for host-specific toxins lie on the cell membrane, there are exceptions. *Helminthosporium maydis* race T produces a toxin which has very rapid effects on mitochondria isolated from susceptible maize plants. Within one minute of exposure to T toxin, ATP levels begin to fall, and the harmful effects on host cells have in this case been attributed to sudden loss of respiratory control.

Non-specific toxins

The discovery of toxins with host-specificity and an ability to incite all of the symptoms associated with infection by a particular pathogen has given a considerable stimulus to the toxigenic theory of disease. It is important to realize, however, that host-specific toxins have so far been identified in only a minority of plant diseases. In many other diseases, toxins account for at least some of the symptoms, but do not seem to be the exclusive determinants of pathogenicity. These compounds are perhaps best regarded as factors contributing to the virulence of a pathogen.

Non-specific toxins have effects on plant species other than the natural host. The bacterium *Pseudomonas tabaci*, for instance, causes wildfire disease in tobacco, but wildfire toxin, which is an amino acid analogue, induces chlorotic symptoms in many other plants. Tentoxin, produced by the fungus *Alternaria alternata*, is a broad-spectrum toxin with activity against gymnosperms, pteridophytes, mosses and green algae as well as a wide range of higher plants. Sensitivity to tentoxin is correlated with binding to a chloroplast fraction and inhibition of photophosphorylation.

In many cases, the precise role of non-specific toxins in a disease is controversial. For instance, the correlation of toxin production with virulence may be questionable; alternaric acid has been detected in lesions on potato leaves caused by *Alternaria solani*, but strains of the pathogen which produce large amounts of this compound *in vitro* are not necessarily highly virulent.

Not all phytotoxic substances produced by pathogens are small molecules. Several compounds implicated in vascular wilt diseases have been shown to be high-molecular-weight polysaccharides or glycopeptides. *Corynebacterium insidiosum*, the causal agent of bacterial wilt in alfalfa, elaborates a large glycopeptide in culture which induces wilt symptoms in bioassays, and which has also been isolated from diseased plants. These substances may impair water flow by virtue of their size. In fact, their toxicity may be related to their molecular weight. Experiments with synthetic polymers have shown that if their mol. wt is $< 50\,000$ they can be transported through the xylem and act in the leaves; if > 50 000 they remain in the xylem and contribute to the physical plugging of the vessels.

The role played by toxins in vascular wilt diseases highlights the difficulty of proving the involvement of any particular compound in pathogenesis. A diverse array of toxic substances has been isolated from the culture filtrates of wilt pathogens, ranging from simple organic acids to highly complex macromolecules. However, after starring briefly in the pathological literature, most of these have subsequently been relegated to, at best, a subsidiary role in disease causation.

Phytoalexins

Earlier in this chapter we saw that following infection the activity of certain biosynthetic pathways is stimulated; as a result, novel compounds which are absent from healthy tissue, or which are present in only trace amounts, accumulate in the host–pathogen complex. Many of these compounds inhibit fungi and bacteria, and may therefore play a part in the host's defence reaction.

The term phytoalexin was first introduced by Muller and Borger in 1940 to describe fungistatic or fungitoxic compounds produced during the hypersensitive response of potato tubers to incompatible races of *Phytophthora infestans*. Since that time it has been shown that many other plant species produce phytoalexins in response to infection, and a number of these have been successfully isolated and characterized. The structures of six are shown in Fig. 8.15.

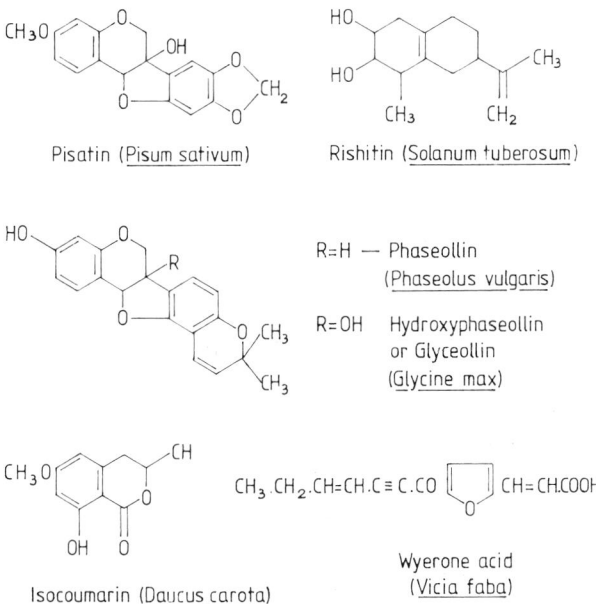

Figure 8.15 Structure and source of several phytoalexins.

All these examples are either from plant storage tissues, or from species of the family Leguminosae. This is merely a reflection of the fact that most of the pioneering work on phytoalexins has been carried out with one or other of these tissue types. It now seems likely that the capacity to produce phytoalexins is widespread amongst plant families. For some time it was believed that the cereals were unable to synthesize phytoalexins, but recent work has shown that barley, oats and rice can all form such compounds.

Legume seed pods provide a particularly convenient system for demonstrating phytoalexin production, as the inner surface (or endocarp) of the seed cavity can be exposed and inoculated without subjecting the tissues to injury. In addition, the endocarp is devoid of cuticle or epidermis, and spore suspensions of fungi or other agents can be placed in direct contact with the tissues. The diffusion of inhibitory compounds into droplets containing various pathogens or non-pathogens can then be studied. If this 'droplet diffusate technique' is applied to pea pods, accumulation of the phytoalexin pisatin starts within 12 hours and reaches a peak after 2–3 days (Fig. 8.16). The concentration of phytoalexin which accumulates shows a linear re-

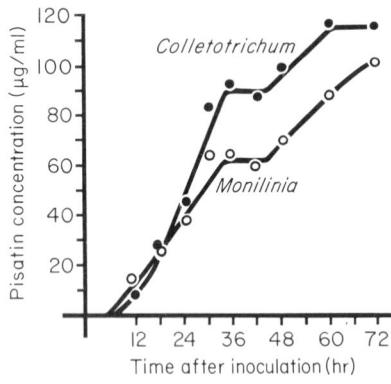

Figure 8.16 Accumulation of pisatin in diffusates following inoculation of pea pod endocarp with two non-pathogens, *Colletotrichum lindemuthianum* and *Monilinia fructicola* (data from Kuć, 1971).

lationship to the amount of inoculum applied (i.e. number of spores), in other words, the more inoculum applied, the more phytoalexin produced. A similar result is obtained with French beans, but in this case the phytoalexin formed is phaseollin.

The detection of phytoalexins in plant tissues rather than drop diffusates relies upon procedures for extracting and purifying the compounds, coupled with an appropriate bioassay to determine their antimicrobial activity. For convenience, these steps are sometimes combined. Figure 8.17 shows a thin-layer chromatography plate which has been used to separate phytoalexins produced by broad bean in response to inoculation with *Botrytis cinerea*. Antifungal compounds have been directly located on the plate by spraying it with spores of a dark-coloured fungus, *Cladosporium herbarum*, suspended in a nutrient solution. The fungus grows all over the plate except where inhibited by these compounds, which therefore show up as clear white areas of silica gel. A further important point should be noted in this

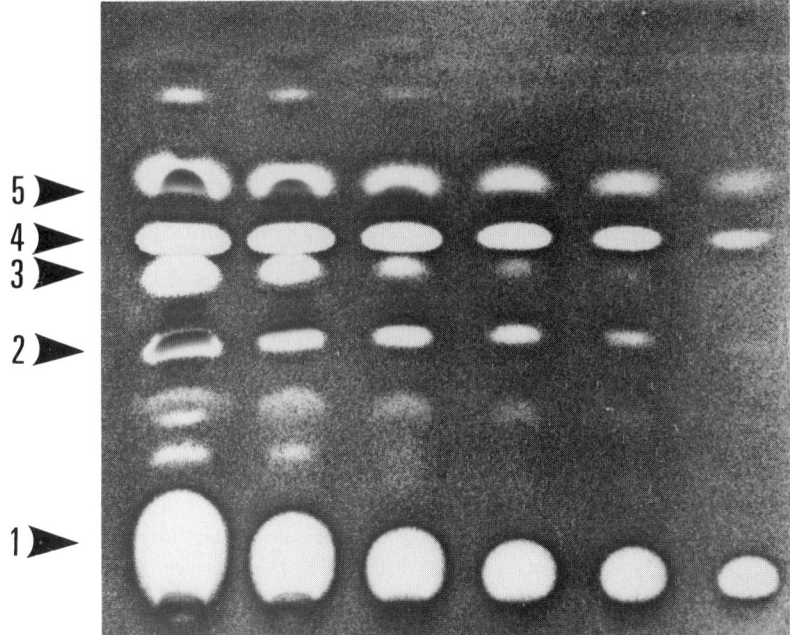

Figure 8.17 Bioassay of phytoalexins produced by broad bean leaves in response to inoculation with the fungus *Botrytis cinerea*. Extracts from 0.4, 0.2, 0.1, 0.05, 0.025 and 0.0125 g of tissue were collected three days after inoculation and separated by thin-layer chromatography. Antifungal compounds were then located by spraying the plate with a spore suspension of the dark-coloured fungus *Cladosporium herbarum*. Phytoalexins identified are (1) wyerone acid, (2) medicarpin, (3) wyerol, (4) wyerone epoxide and (5) wyerone. (Photograph from Hargreaves *et al.*, 1977.)

figure. Plants challenged with micro-organisms often produce several phytoalexins which may be structurally related, even isomeric forms, or alternatively produced by quite different biosynthetic pathways.

Phytoalexins and resistance

Evaluation of the role played by phytoalexins in disease resistance has raised a number of questions.

1. Are these compounds specific in the sense that they are only produced in response to non-pathogens or non-virulent races of a pathogen? In actual fact, phytoalexins are formed in response to a wide variety of agents. Pisatin, for instance, is induced by metabolic inhibitors such as heavy metals, by cyanide, and by compounds which affect DNA, as well as by microbial agents. Infection by viruses induces phaseollin production in beans. The induction of phytoalexins is, therefore, relatively non-specific, and they can be regarded as stress metabolites rather than highly specific resistance factors. In fact, phytoalexins are now defined as 'substances formed by host tissue in response to injury, physiological stimuli, infectious agents or their products, that accumulate to levels which inhibit the growth of micro-organisms'.

2. Are phytoalexins selective, in other words are they more toxic to non-pathogens than to pathogens? Although compounds such as pisatin are essentially weak antibiotics with a broad spectrum of activity towards many micro-organisms, there is evidence that non-pathogens are generally more sensitive to phytoalexins than pathogens. For instance, phaseollin has a fungistatic effect on *Monilinia fructicola*, a non-pathogen of beans, at concentrations as low as 3 μg/ml whereas 50 μg/ml are required to have a similar effect on *Colletotrichum lindemuthianum*, which causes bean anthracnose. This difference probably reflects the differing abilities of the two fungi to degrade and detoxify the phytoalexin.

3. Are phytoalexins produced at the right place at the right time at a concentration sufficient to account for cessation of growth of the pathogen? This is the critical question but it is also the hardest to answer. It is extremely difficult to estimate the concentration of a compound at the infection site itself, but this is where the success or failure of a potential pathogen is determined. The *in vivo* concentration of a phytoalexin may in fact be at a level where even fairly subtle differences in the sensitivity of different micro-organisms would prove critical. Similarly, the relative rate at which a phytoalexin accumulates in a particular host–pathogen combination is probably more important than the final concentration achieved. Figure 8.18 shows that phaseollin accumulates earlier in beans reacting hypersensitively to *Colletotrichum lindemuthianum* than in beans infected by a compatible race of the same pathogen. Although higher levels eventually accumulate in the compatible combination, the lesions are already well established and the pathogen has, in effect, escaped.

A convincing answer to this last question demands careful correlations between the growth rate of an invading organism and the amount of phytoa-

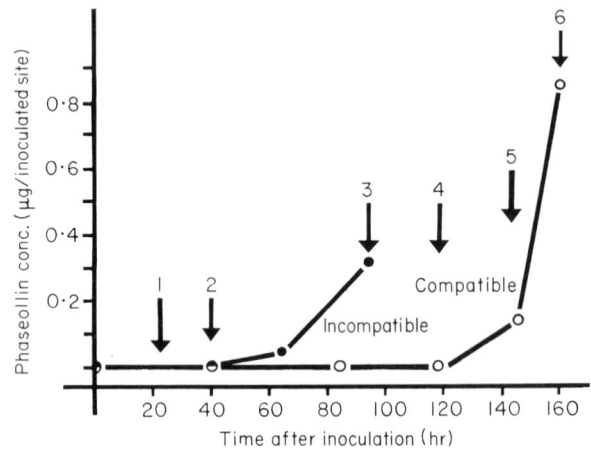

Figure 8.18 Accumulation of phaseollin in beans inoculated with compatible and incompatible races of anthracrose fungus. Stage 1 = appressorium formation, 2 = hypersensitive response visible, 3 = hypersensitive response complete, 4 = 1% lesions in compatible combination, 5 = 80% lesions, 6 = 100% lesions. (Data from Bailey & Deverall, 1971.)

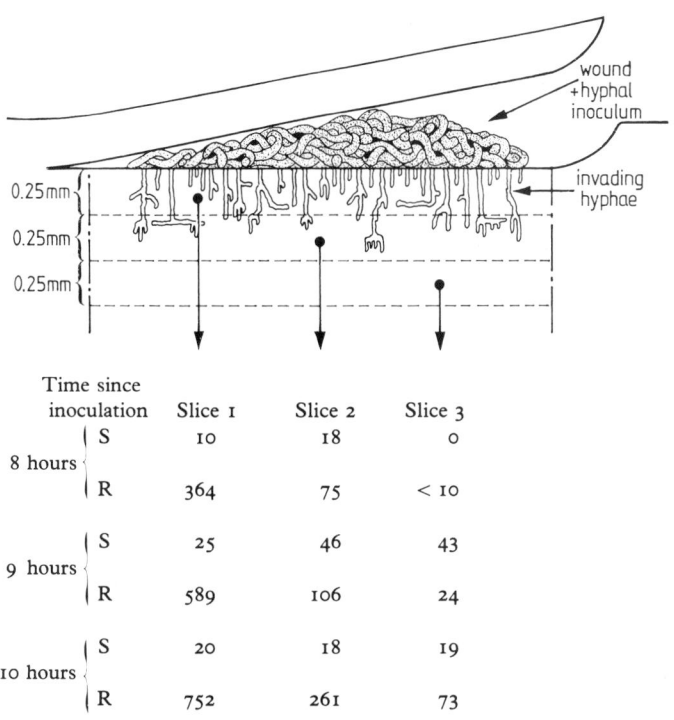

Time since inoculation		Slice 1	Slice 2	Slice 3
8 hours	S	10	18	0
	R	364	75	< 10
9 hours	S	25	46	43
	R	589	106	24
10 hours	S	20	18	19
	R	752	261	73

Figure 8.19 Accumulation of the phytoalexin glyceollin in soybean hypocotyls susceptible (S) and resistant (R) to race 1 of *Phytophthora megasperma* var. *sojae*. The inoculation and sampling method shown was used to obtain the time-course data presented below. In the susceptible cultivar the fungus is colonizing slice 3 by 10 hours after inoculation, whereas in the resistant cultivar it remains restricted to the top two slices. The level of glyceollin required to inhibit hyphal growth is approximately 200 μmol/ml. (Data from Yoshikawa *et al.*, 1978.)

lexin present at specific tissue sites. One of the most intensively studied systems in this respect is the interaction of the fungus *Phytophthora megasperma* var. *sojae* (often abbreviated to Pms) with soybean. The cultivar Harosoy is susceptible to race 1 of Pms, while the cultivar Harosoy 63 carries a single gene for resistance. Expression of race-specific resistance in H63 is accompanied by accumulation of the phytoalexin glyceollin (see Fig. 8.15). For the first eight hours following inoculation the growth rate of the fungus is similar in hypocotyls of both cultivars. Growth is arrested in H63 between eight and nine hours after inoculation, but it continues unchecked in the susceptible cultivar. Trying to attribute this difference in growth rates to the accumulation of glyceollin is problematical as only trace amounts can be detected in resistant hypocotyls ten hours after inoculation. Toxic levels of the phytoalexin appear to build up in intact hypocotyls too late to account for inhibition of the pathogen.

Using a more exacting sampling procedure, however, a quite different story emerges (Fig. 8.19). Analysis of thin slices of hypocotyl tissue taken directly below the inoculation site shows that the concentration of glyceollin in the resistant cultivar is more than sufficient to inhibit the fungus by the time growth is checked. The failure of the pathogen to colonize resistant hypocotyl tissues can therefore be directly attributed to phytoalexin accumulation.

Experiments such as these argue strongly for a causal role for phytoalexins in disease resistance. In the Pms–soybean interaction it now seems clear that race-specific resistance is due to the *de novo* synthesis of messenger RNA and protein, leading to accumulation of an inhibitory concentration of an antifungal compound. For many other systems the current evidence is less convincing. Several studies have suggested that phytoalexin production is a consequence, rather than a cause, of resistance. Accumulation of rishitin in potato tissues undergoing a resistance reaction to *Phytophthora infestans* appears to be a secondary effect. It should also be remembered that the phytoalexins so far characterized have little influence on the resistance of plants to bacteria, and no effect on viruses.

An alternative approach which promises to clarify the whole problem of phytoalexins and resistance is to investigate how infection by a microorganism incites the production of inhibitory compounds by the host. This will be discussed further in Chapter 9.

Growth regulators

No discussion of low-molecular-weight compounds in plant disease would be complete without mention of plant growth regulators. Many pathogens cause characteristic malformations of host tissues (Fig. 7.17), and these developmental abnormalities are due to alterations in the hormonal balance of the plant. Four classes of compound are known to be involved: auxins, such as indole-3-acetic acid (IAA), gibberellins, cytokinins and the volatile hormone ethylene.

Evaluation of the role played by individual growth regulators in pathogenesis is complex because their physiological effects in many cases overlap, and normal plant growth and development is determined by the integrated action of several types of hormone rather than by changes in the concentration of a single compound.

A typical feature of many diseases causing growth abnormalities is an increase in the concentration of one or more hormonal compounds in the host–pathogen complex. Hyperauxiny, or the accumulation of unusually high concentrations of IAA, is found in a variety of diseases, including crown gall, smut of maize and vascular wilts. There are three possible explanations for this increase in auxin concentrations:

1 Synthesis of auxin by the host is stimulated. There is good evidence that the abnormal amounts of auxin found in crown gall tumours are produced by the host.

2 The auxin is secreted by the pathogen. *Ustilago maydis, Fusarium oxysporum, Taphrina deformans* and several other pathogens produce IAA in culture.

3 The rate of degradation of auxin is suppressed, due to a reduction in the

activity of the enzyme IAA oxidase. In tobacco infected by TMV or *Pseudomonas solanacearum*, IAA oxidase activity is depressed. Inhibition of the enzyme by phenolic compounds which accumulate in diseased tissues has been demonstrated.

Of course, more than one of these explanations may be involved. In tobacco infected by *P. solanacearum,* the early increase in auxin has been attributed to synthesis by the host, while in the later stages of infection synthesis by the bacterium and a reduction in the rate of IAA degradation both seem to contribute as well.

Gibberellins are to some extent synonymous with plant disease as this class of physiologically active compounds was first identified in culture filtrates of the fungus *Gibberella fujikuroi*, the causal agent of 'foolish seedling' disease of rice. In this disease infected plants outgrow normal plants and become weak and spindly. This symptom is due to the secretion of gibberellins by the pathogen in the host. The part played by gibberellins in other diseases is, however, less clear. The stunting caused by some viruses can be reversed by applying exogenous gibberellins, suggesting that the reduced growth of these plants might be due to a decreased gibberellin content.

Abnormal cell division, leading to tumours and galls, is another common symptom of disease. As cytokinins participate in the control of cell division it is hardly surprising that these compounds should be implicated in cases involving uncontrolled cell multiplication. Peach leaves affected by *Taphrina deformans* exhibit higher cytokinin activity than healthy leaves. Chromatographic analysis of leaf extracts has shown that three cytokinins found in healthy leaves are more active in diseased leaves. An additional cytokinin not present in healthy leaves has also been detected. It appears that this compound is secreted by the pathogen. Peach leaf curl symptoms cannot however be entirely attributed to changes in cytokinins, as the level of IAA also increases in diseased leaves.

Ethylene

From time to time in this chapter we have mentioned the broad similarities between the metabolic changes characteristic of infected tissues and those observed in plants subjected to other types of stress. These similarities suggest that plant tissues exhibit a common stress response to a variety of injurious agents. The actual trigger or 'master switch' which sets off the whole chain of metabolic events following stress is not known, but ethylene has been suggested as a possible inducer for a number of reasons. In the first place it is volatile and active at very low concentrations. Secondly, it has a wide variety of physiological effects, including the activation or synthesis of enzymes such as PAL and peroxidase. It may also act as a synergist, for example by increasing the severity of symptoms induced by toxins. Thirdly, increased amounts of ethylene are evolved from plant tissues infected by fungi, bacteria and viruses, as well as by injured tissues. Figure 8.20

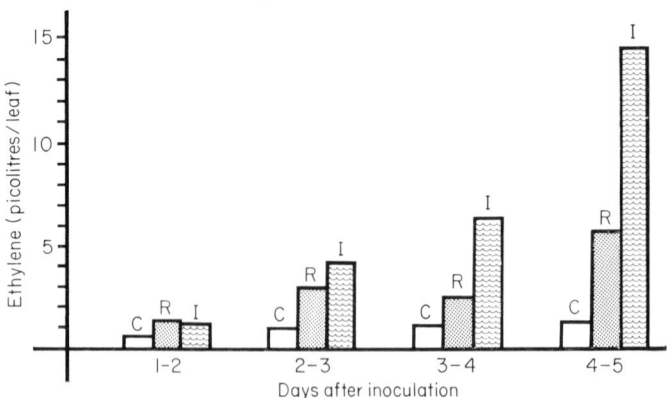

Figure 8.20 Ethylene evolution from wheat leaves infected by *Puccinia graminis*.
C = uninoculated controls, R = resistant inoculated, I = non-resistant inoculated. (Data from
Daly *et al.*, 1970.)

shows the increase in ethylene evolution from wheat leaves inoculated with
Puccinia graminis; both incompatible and compatible combinations evolve
higher amounts of ethylene than control leaves, but the most dramatic increase occurs in the compatible interaction at the time when the pathogen
starts to sporulate. A similar pattern is seen in barley leaves infected by
Erysiphe graminis. In this case, however, there is some evidence that a
short-lived burst of ethylene evolution occurs early in the incompatible
combination. The idea that ethylene might be involved in resistance has
received more conclusive support from studies on sweet potato tissue. Resistance to *Ceràtocystis fimbriata* can be induced by exposing previously
non-resistant sweet potato tissue to ethylene. This induction is accompanied
by increases in the activity of peroxidase and polyphenol oxidase. Due to its
volatile nature, ethylene might diffuse from initial infection sites to surrounding tissues and initiate metabolic changes which contribute to the
subsequent limitation of the infection. However, like many other problems
in the biochemistry of host–pathogen interaction it is not yet clear whether
ethylene is a primary factor in triggering metabolic changes or is merely
produced as a result of these changes.

FURTHER READING

General texts

WHEELER H. (1975) *Plant Pathogenesis*. Springer Verlag, Berlin.
    A concise and stimulating introduction to physiological aspects of plant–pathogen interac-
    tions.
WOOD R.K.S. & GRANITI A. eds (1976) *Specificity in Plant Diseases*. Plenum Press, New York.
    Proceedings of a conference, including some lively discussion sessions.

Reviews and original articles

BATEMAN D.F. & BASHAM H.G. (1976) Degradation of plant cell walls and membranes by
    microbial enzymes. In *Encyclopedia of Plant Physiology*, Vol. IV, *Physiological Plant Path-
    ology* (eds Heitefuss R. & Williams P.H.), pp. 316–355. Springer Verlag, Berlin.

BELL A.A. (1981) Biochemical mechanisms of disease resistance. *Annual Review of Plant Physiology* **32**, 21–81.

BRIAN P.W. (1978) Hormones in healthy and diseased plants. *Proceedings of the Royal Society of London Series B* **200**, 231–43.

DALY J.M. (1976) Some aspects of host–pathogen interactions. In *Encyclopedia of Plant Physiology*, Vol. IV., *Physiological Plant Pathology* (eds Heitefuss R. & Williams P.H.), pp. 27–50. Springer Verlag, Berlin.

HISLOP E.C., HOAD G.V. & ARCHER S.A. (1973) The involvement of ethylene in plant disease. In *Fungal Pathogenicity and the Plant's Response* (eds Byrde R.J.W. & Cutting C.V.), pp. 87–113. Academic Press, London.

MERLO D.J. (1978) Crown gall—a unique disease. In *Plant Disease* Vol. III (eds Horsfall J.G. & Cowling E.B.), pp. 201–213. Academic Press, New York.

SAMBORSKI D.J., ROHRINGER R. & KIM W.K. (1978) Transcription and translation in diseased plants. In *Plant Disease* Vol. III (eds Horsfall J.G. & Cowling E.B.), pp. 375–390. Academic Press, New York.

WALTON J.D. *et al.* (1979) Reduction of adenosine triphosphate levels in susceptible maize mesophyll protoplasts by *Helminthosporium maydis* race T toxin. *Plant Physiology* **63**, 806–10.

YODER O.C. (1980) Toxins in pathogenesis. *Annual Review of Phytopathology* **18**, 103–129.

YOSHIKAWA M., YAMAUCHI K. & MASAGO H. (1978) *De novo* messenger RNA and protein synthesis are required for phytoalexin-mediated disease resistance in soybean hypocotyls. *Plant Physiology* **61**, 314–17.

YOSHIKAWA M., YAMAUCHI K. & MASAGO H. (1978) Glyceollin: its role in restricting fungal growth in resistant soybean hypocotyls infected with *Phytophthora megasperma* var. *sojae*. *Physiological Plant Pathology* **12**, 73–82.

9 Host–pathogen specificity

> "We cannot remind ourselves too often that disease is a relatively rare phenomenon and that particular pathogens are able to parasitize only a very small proportion of the plants available to them."
>
> R.K.S. WOOD (1919–)

Why certain micro-organisms are able to cause disease, whilst the majority cannot, is currently a crucial question in pathology. Despite advances in our understanding of molecular aspects of plant–microbe interactions, no satisfactory answer to this question has yet emerged. Specificity involves not only the factors determining virulence in the pathogen but also those conferring resistance on the host. We have already seen in previous chapters that pathogen virulence and host resistance may both be determined by more than one factor and the interaction between them is complex rather than simple.

Understanding specificity is important for both practical and conceptual reasons. First and foremost, a complete analysis of the problem will allow us to devise more precise and reliable ways of controlling plant disease, either through specifically tailored chemical compounds or through better techniques for breeding and deploying resistant crops. In addition, insights into the nature of host–pathogen specificity are likely to prove relevant to compatibility phenomena in other biological systems, such as the pollen–stigma interaction and tissue rejection in transplantation surgery.

TYPES OF SPECIFICITY

It should be appreciated at the outset that host–pathogen specificity involves several separate and probably different phenomena. In the first place there is the absolute distinction between parasitic organisms and those which are unable to attack living hosts under any circumstances. Parasitic microbes must possess properties which enable them to grow successfully in plant tissues, but surprisingly little is known about why this ability to infect living plants is the exception rather than the rule.

Amongst parasites there are those with a wide host range embracing diverse taxonomic groups and those restricted to one or a few host species.

Even with a versatile parasite, however, the majority of plant species will be resistant. Our explanation of specificity must include this distinction between host and non-host species.

Further degrees of specificity are seen in parasites with a narrow range of potential hosts, where specialization even within that range often occurs. For instance, cereal rust and powdery mildew fungi exist as distinct form species on particular cereal hosts. Even greater specificity may be seen at this level in pathogen races distinguished only by their reaction types on a series of host cultivars which differ in one or a few resistance genes. This extreme specificity is described in genetic terms by the gene-for-gene theory (see p. 30).

Yet another form of specificity, often overlooked, is where a parasitic microbe is restricted to particular host tissues or organs. Such tissue specificity is alluded to in many common names for pathogens, for example root rot, leaf mould and vascular wilt. Once again, the factors controlling these patterns of colonization are poorly understood.

No single model of host–pathogen specificity seems likely to explain all these phenomena. The factors enabling a non-specialized parasite to attack a diversity of host species may be different from those enabling a new mutant race of a pathogen to infect a previously resistant host cultivar. Does this mean that plant pathologists should abandon their search for a unifying concept in host–pathogen interaction? Certainly not, for while the specific mechanisms controlling the outcome of each interaction may differ, there may well be a common framework underlying all these different plant–microbe confrontations.

TYPES OF HOST RESISTANCE

Plants possess a number of different resistance mechanisms which can all be classified as either PASSIVE or ACTIVE (Fig. 9.1). Passive resistance mechanisms are best visualized as anatomical or chemical barricades preventing establishment of the pathogen. These barricades are present prior to infection and therefore represent a constitutive feature of the host. In contrast, active resistance mechanisms are induced by challenge with a microorganism and cannot be detected in healthy plants prior to inoculation.

In addition to the mechanisms listed in Fig. 9.1, a quite different type of resistance may occur. In natural populations, plants might possess "avoidance mechanisms" whereby they escape contact with the pathogen by growing in an environment unfavourable for the latter or by completing their life cycle during periods when the pathogen is inactive. As this situation does not involve any confrontation between the two partners it will not be considered further in our discussion.

Passive anatomical features, such as the cuticle and bark, represent highly effective barriers to infection. Such physical obstacles are often supplemented by preformed chemical inhibitors. Plants synthesize an impressive array of secondary metabolites and many of these are toxic to potential

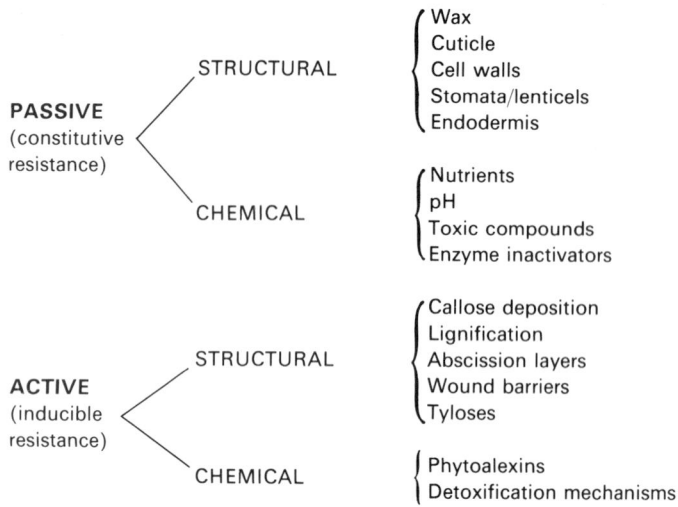

Figure 9.1   Classification of the main resistance mechanisms in green plants.

pests and pathogens. In addition to the fungitoxic phenols discussed in Chapter 8, alkaloids, glucosides, tannins and resins have all been implicated in disease resistance. Resins, for example, are known to increase the resistance of conifers to attack by wood-rotting fungi. Although all these inhibitors are present prior to infection, they may not in fact be effective until released through tissue damage or degradation by enzymes. Glucosides which are not themselves toxic break down to release highly toxic aglycones; any pathogen producing the necessary glucosidase enzyme may therefore contribute to its own downfall! Other preformed host components, while not toxic to the pathogen itself, may inhibit some essential step in pathogenesis. Pectolytic enzymes, which facilitate the colonization of host tissues by various pathogens, can be inactivated by specific glycoproteins located in the host cell wall. This discovery has strengthened the view that the composition and structure of plant cell walls determines the relative success of many necrotrophic pathogens.

Should the passive defences of the plant be breached or overcome by the pathogen, then active resistance mechanisms come into play. The participation of active metabolism in resistance mechanisms may be deduced from experiments in which plants have been treated with narcotics during infection. Such treatment often sufficiently lowers host resistance to allow rapid colonization by the pathogen. Active mechanisms may also be classified as structural or chemical (Fig. 9.1). In practice, however, the distinction between these categories may be more apparent than real. Thus, the development of wound barriers and synthesis of phytoalexins both represent complementary aspects of an overall response to the pathogen. Similarly, precursors of structural polymers, such as lignin, are toxic and may act as inhibitors within the host–pathogen complex. We have already seen that one of the most dramatic examples of active resistance, the hypersensitive response, involves several components, including accumulation of phytoalexins, cell wall alterations and wound repair mechanisms in adjacent tissues.

Four main features of host response to infection emerge:
(1) Synthesis of new macromolecules
e.g. nucleic acids, proteins, polysaccharides.
(2) Acceleration of metabolism
e.g. increased respiration, more mitochondria.
(3) Alterations in the activity or direction of metabolic pathways
e.g. shikimic acid pathway.
(4) Production of abnormal or stress metabolites
e.g. phytoalexins.

The sum total of these changes is the creation of a cellular environment which inhibits the establishment of the pathogen.

INDUCTION OF HOST RESISTANCE MECHANISMS

An active resistance mechanism, by definition, requires a system for triggering the response. At its simplest such a system must comprise a host receptor site and some component of the pathogen which interacts with this site and 'switches on' the response.

Elicitors

Experiments on the induction of phytoalexin accumulation in plants have provided some clues as to how active resistance might be triggered. It has been repeatedly shown that fungal-culture filtrates or extracts of microbial cell walls can induce phytoalexin accumulation in plant tissues. The compounds responsible are known as ELICITORS. Elicitors are chemically diverse; the first to be isolated, Monilicolin A from the fungus *Monilinia fructicola*, is a small polypeptide. Most other elicitors so far characterized have turned out to be either polysaccharides or glycoproteins (Table 9.1). Attempts to purify them to a single active fraction indicate that they are heterogeneous in size, and this, together with their chemical similarity to components of microbial cell walls, suggests that the active molecules are fragments of natural wall polymers. Another notable feature of elicitors is their extremely high activity; the glucans isolated from Pms induce glyceollin synthesis in soybean if present at concentrations as low as 10^{-12} molar.

The important conclusion to be drawn at this point is that the surface layers of fungi and bacteria contain components which can activate plant defence reactions.

What part do elicitors play in the determination of host–pathogen speci-

Table 9.1 Some biotic phytoalexin elicitors (adapted from Wade, unpublished).

Source organism	Chemical nature	Mol. wt	Activity
FUNGAL PATHOGENS			
Monilinia fructicola	Polypeptide	*c.* 8000	Induces phaseollin in bean
Phytophthora megasperma sojae (Pms)	Glucan	$2 \times 10^3 - 10^5$	Induces glyceollin in soybean
	Glycoprotein	—	Specifically induces glyceollin in soybean
Colletotrichum lindemuthianum	Glucan	$1 - 5 \times 10^6$	Induces hypersensitivity and phaseollin in bean
FUNGAL NON-PATHOGENS			
Saccharomyces cerevisiae	Glucan	Heterogeneous	Induces phytoalexins in soybean, bean, potato, etc
BACTERIAL PATHOGEN			
Pseudomonas glycinea	Glycoprotein	—	Specifically induces glyceollin in soybean

ficity? There are two possibilities. The first is that these compounds, while playing a key role in general resistance, are non-specific in action. Plant cells may be able to recognize a wide variety of foreign microbes on the basis of one or a few surface polymers common to them all. According to this view, elicitors are part of a non-specific recognition mechanism and therefore incidental to the factors controlling, for instance, race specificity. The alternative view is that elicitors determine race-specificity. Subtle differences in the surface molecules of pathogen races would then account for the induction or non-induction of host resistance. In a gene-for-gene system, an elicitor might be the specific product of a pathogen avirulence gene which interacts with the host resistance gene.

At present, the weight of evidence favours the former view. For instance, the glucan elicitors from different races of Pms are all equally effective in stimulating glyceollin synthesis in soybeans. Studies on other pathogens have also failed to detect differences in the activity of elicitors from virulent and avirulent races. Furthermore, effective elicitors can be isolated from non-pathogens, including the yeast *Saccharomyces cerevisiae* (Table 9.1). There is, in addition, a conceptual difficulty to be overcome in regarding elicitors as specificity factors. Some pathogens exist in the form of a very large number of races, and specific elicitors would, therefore, need to be present in numerous subtle structural permutations.

In spite of these objections, some workers have claimed to have isolated elicitors which parallel the specificity of the intact pathogen. Glycoproteins extracted from different races of Pms have exhibited differential activity on soybean cultivars and might, therefore, be specific determinants of resistance in this system. One unresolved difficulty here is that the glucan elicitors from Pms are much more effective as elicitors than these glycoproteins.

In a natural interaction, any differential effects based on the latter would surely be masked by a flood of non-specifically induced phytoalexin! However, the glycoproteins remain of interest, particularly as it has been shown that treatment with glycoproteins from avirulent races of Pms can protect soybean cultivars against subsequent infection by virulent races. This effect could not be explained in terms of specific phytoalexin accumulation as the glycoproteins concerned had little elicitor activity. One possible explanation is that they somehow modulate the action of the non-specific glucan elicitors.

Thus, the discovery of phytoalexin elicitors has raised almost as many questions as it has solved. At one extreme, elicitors may be regarded as being no different from the many other physical and chemical agents which induce phytoalexin accumulation (see Chapter 8). However, recent studies have suggested that biotic and abiotic agents may increase phytoalexin levels in quite different ways. Phytoalexin accumulation can reflect either increased synthesis of the compound or a lower rate of breakdown by the plant itself. Comparisons between glucan elicitors from fungi and abiotic agents, such as heavy-metal ions, showed that the former stimulate biosynthesis of phytoalexin, while the latter mainly act by inhibiting degradation. However, this conclusion has been challenged by other scientists who could find little difference in the rate of synthesis using either type of elicitor.

Finally, we should note that arguments about phytoalexin elicitors and host–pathogen specificity presuppose that differential accumulation of phytoalexin is the major determinant of disease resistance. As we have seen earlier, this is probably not the case in all host–pathogen systems. Elicitors of other host responses, such as lignification, have also been described. No doubt there must be elicitors of all the different types of active defence mechanisms. In addition, plant cells can produce their own endogenous elicitors; when bean tissues are killed by freezing and thawing, a factor diffuses into adjacent live cells and triggers phaseollin accumulation. This observation is consistent with the idea that hypersensitive cell death may itself play a part in switching on the plant's defence systems.

Susceptibility as an induced state

There is an opposite, and in some ways more logical, approach to the problem of host–pathogen specificity. Since susceptibility is the exception rather than the rule and the majority of plant–microbe combinations are incompatible, perhaps we should be looking for the special properties of the susceptible interaction. In particular, how does the successful pathogen confound the host's recognition system or, alternatively, suppress the normal resistance response? According to this view susceptibility, rather than resistance, is the induced state, and should thus provide the key to understanding the mechanism of specificity.

This argument may be persuasive, but is there any evidence to support it? In actual fact, quite a large body of experimental data favours the idea. Most of this evidence concerns the suppression of host resistance by a virulent pathogen, rather than strategies for bypassing the recognition system itself.

SUPPRESSION OF HOST RESISTANCE RESPONSES

Experiments with several biotrophic fungi have shown that pre-inoculation with a compatible pathogen can lower the resistance of the host plant to subsequent inoculation with an incompatible pathogen. For instance, if barley leaves are inoculated with *Erysiphe graminis* f.sp. *hordei* and two days later the developing colonies are peeled off and replaced by spores of the normally incompatible wheat form of the fungus, *E. graminis* f.sp. *tritici*, some growth and development of the latter will occur. Similarly, rust species normally incapable of infecting non-host leaves may penetrate and produce haustoria in tissues adjacent to colonies of a compatible rust species. Observations like these have been interpreted as showing that a virulent pathogen can in some way 'condition' host tissues to accept another pathogen, which in the usual course of events would fail to establish. The obvious conclusion is that the host's response is inhibited or impaired by the virulent pathogen.

More direct evidence that pathogens may be able to suppress host resistance comes from work on *Phytophthora infestans*. Water-soluble glucans from compatible races of the fungus have been shown to suppress the hypersensitive response of potato protoplasts exposed to hyphal-wall components of the pathogen. As the activity showed to some extent the same specificity as the pathogen-race–host-cultivar combination, these glucans could be the determinants of specificity in this system. According to this hypothesis, resistance is triggered by all races of the pathogen, but specific suppressors from compatible races are able to curtail the response. Thus resistance results from an interaction between host cells and non-specific elicitors, whereas a dual interaction with both elicitors and specific suppressors leads to susceptibility.

There are a few reports that pathogens may also actively suppress phytoalexin production. Further evidence is, however, required to confirm whether such an interplay between the elicitation and suppression of host resistance mechanisms can explain specificity.

DESTRUCTION OF THE HOST'S RESISTANCE RESPONSE

An alternative strategy to the suppression of host resistance is for the pathogen to kill host cells so quickly that no effective response can be mounted. It need hardly be added that this option is only open to necrotrophic pathogens.

174

When broad beans are inoculated with *Botytis cinerea*, the fungus is restricted to small necrotic lesions; with the closely related species *B. fabae*, the fungus continues to colonize leaf tissues, giving rise to much larger, spreading lesions. If one measures the level of the predominant broad-bean phytoalexin wyerone acid (see Fig. 8.15) accumulating in these different types of lesion, an interesting contrast emerges (Fig. 9.2). In the case of the weakly pathogenic *B. cinerea* the amount of phytoalexin continues to increase over the first three days to reach a level sufficient to account for inhibition of the pathogen. With the aggressive *B. fabae*, wyerone acid starts

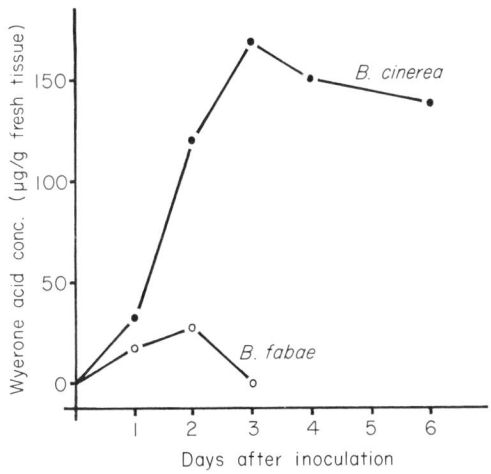

Figure 9.2 Accumulation of wyerone acid in leaf tissues and droplets containing spores of either *Botrytis cinerea* or *B. fabae* placed on leaves of *Vicia faba* (data from Hargreaves *et al.*, 1977).

to accumulate but subsequently declines to a level where it can no longer be detected. Two factors seem to determine this difference. First, *B. fabae* is less sensitive to the phytoalexin than *B. cinerea*. This is critical in the early stages of infection when the pathogen must establish itself in the face of a mounting host response. Secondly, *B. fabae* kills host cells much more rapidly than *B. cinerea*. The lethal factors have not yet been identified, but they may be pectolytic enzymes. Once it has gained a foothold, the aggressive pathogen kills cells around the lesion sufficiently quickly to limit phytoalexin production. In fact, as the lesions expand, the fungus is able to metabolize the relatively small amounts of phytoalexin to which it is then exposed.

Other host–pathogen interactions in which the death of host cells seems to be a prerequisite for susceptibility include those involving host-specific toxins. Virulence in these systems is correlated with production of a toxin which specifically kills cells in the susceptible host (see Chapter 8). No doubt the very rapid membrane damage and other pathological changes leading to cell death again pre-empt an effective host response.

It should be noted that the examples outlined in this section represent the converse of hypersensitivity, where rapid host cell death is a feature of the resistant combination.

A MODEL

These current concepts concerning determination of host–pathogen specificity are summarized in Fig. 9.3. The model is, of necessity, an oversimplification, as it emphasizes hypersensitivity and phytoalexin production to the exclusion of other components of resistance. In addition,

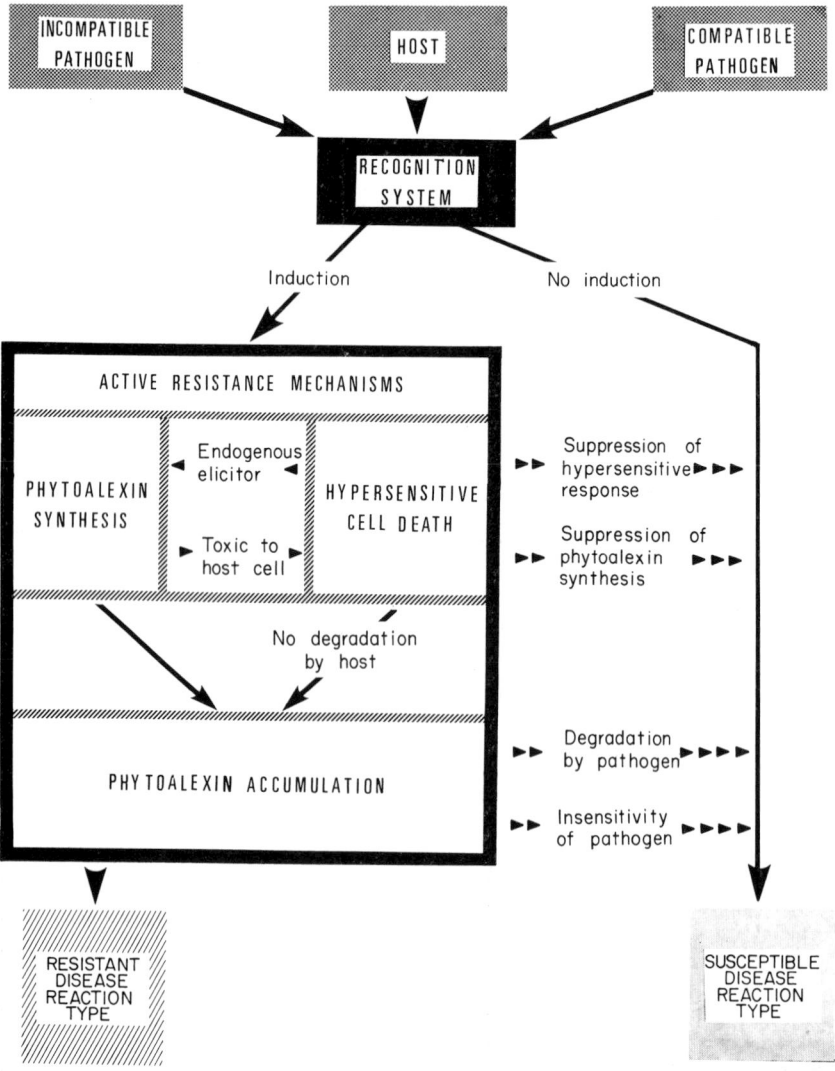

Figure 9.3 A model based on active resistance mechanisms illustrating possible sequences of events leading to resistance or susceptibility.

we make no attempt in our model to weight the various interrelated steps leading to resistance or susceptibility. We have seen that evidence exists for each of the processes outlined in the model. However, the initial recognition step and its connection with resistance mechanisms remain a black box.

THE RECOGNITION MECHANISM

We suggested earlier that the successful pathogen might be the one which is capable of penetrating the host without inducing a resistance response. Put simply, the pathogen bypasses the recognition system that normally alerts the plant to the presence of a foreign organism.

One possibility, already established in animal parasitology, is that the invading organism actually mimics the molecular composition of the host and is therefore sufficiently well disguised to go unnoticed. Although plants do not possess an immunological system comparable to that of animals (see later in this chapter) there is nevertheless some tentative evidence that pathogenic bacteria and fungi share common antigens with their plant hosts. Work with flax cultivars and the rust fungus *Melampsora lini* has shown that compatible races have a greater antigenic affinity with the host than incompatible races. As yet, however, the precise role played by these antigens has not been established.

In biological processes as diverse as fertilization, cell adhesion during morphogenesis and lymphocyte activation by antigens, recognition involves the specific interaction of complementary surface macromolecules. A carbohydrate-binding protein known as a LECTIN, present in the outer membrane or cell envelope of one partner, recognizes specific sugar moieties in glycoproteins or polysaccharides on the surface of the other partner. A similar type of molecular recognition may also be the first event in plant–microbe interactions. We have already seen that some elicitors of host resistance responses are structural polymers located in the cell walls of fungi. In addition, plant cell walls are known to contain lectins with an affinity for various carbohydrates or amino sugars, such as are found in chitin. These molecules might therefore be able to discriminate between different chemical structures specific to the cell surfaces of different micro-organisms.

Experimental evidence in support of such a hypothesis has come mainly from studies on the interactions of bacteria with plant cells. If one infiltrates leaves with a suspension of incompatible bacteria, a hypersensitive response, characterized by rapid host cell collapse and restriction of the bacterial population, takes place (see page 119). In these incompatible lesions, the bacteria quickly become attached to host cells and are then enveloped in a granular or fibrillar matrix. By contrast, compatible bacteria are not entrapped by host cells and continue to multiply freely in the intercellular fluid, causing disintegration of cell walls and eventual destruction of host tissues. Work with several bacterial pathogens, in particular *Pseudomonas solanacearum*, has shown that differences in the lipopolysaccharide outer membrane of the bacterium control binding. Furthermore, a lectin isolated from potato cells specifically agglutinates avirulent isolates of the bacterium, while virulent isolates remain in suspension. Thus it appears that avirulent isolates are recognized and bound by cell wall proteins capable of distinguishing bacterial lipopolysaccharide.

In the example just described, binding to host cells is a feature of incompatible combinations. This is in direct contrast to interactions involving two other closely related bacteria, *Rhizobium* and *Agrobacterium*, where binding by the host cell seems to be a prerequisite for successful infection. Studies on the nodulation of legume roots by different strains of *Rhizobium* have, again, suggested that host lectins may play a part in the recognition mechanism, although one should note that the lectins concerned have usually been isolated from seeds rather than roots. With *Agrobacterium tumefaciens*, attachment to a wound site is the first step in tumour induction; in this case the recognition sites seem to be present in the pectic substances of the host cell middle lamella and are probably polysaccharides rather than proteins. A relatively non-specific recognition mechanism involving polymers common to many different plant species would be consistent with the extremely wide host range of this bacterial pathogen. After initial attachment, the bacteria synthesize cellulose microfibrils which anchor them to the host cell surface (Fig. 9.4) and trap additional bacteria. Transfer of the Ti plasmid to the host cell then takes place, by a mechanism as yet unknown.

While the precise molecular details of these recognition systems remain open to debate, they all seem to fit the general hypothesis that the primary interaction is between surface components capable of distinguishing rather subtle differences in chemical structure. However, even if these models are confirmed, we still have little idea how such a recognition step might activate the defence reaction itself. The nature of the signal linking surface recognition to the metabolic changes which underlie a resistance response remains a mystery.

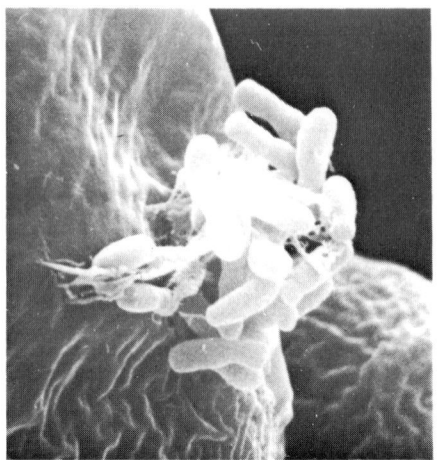

Figure 9.4 Cluster of *Agrobacterium tumefaciens* cells attached to the surface of an isolated plant cell. Note the cellulose fibrils anchoring the bacteria to each other and to the plant cell surface. (Photograph by courtesy of L.J. Seed.)

SPECIFICITY AND PLANT VIRUSES

The problem of host specificity of viruses is unique, as successful reproduction of these pathogens depends upon a precise sequence of molecular events. Thus, the virus must gain entry to the host cell, the nucleic acid must be released from its protein coat, translated and replicated, and new particles must then be assembled. In addition, continuous spread of the virus to other cells and tissues is necessary if systemic colonization of the host is to occur. In theory, specificity might be controlled at any of these steps in the infection cycle. For instance, the lack of appropriate host subunits necessary to form a functional replicase enzyme might prevent more copies of viral nucleic acid being produced. This notion presupposes the necessity of a highly specific 'molecular fit' between host and virus.

In practice, however, factors other than intracellular molecular affinity may well be of greater significance. The need for an appropriate vector to transmit infection adds a further dimension to the equation of virus specificity. The relationships of the virus with the vector and the vector with the host population may limit the host range of a virus to a greater degree than the ability of a pathogen to replicate in host cells. Mechanical inoculation of viruses that are usually transmitted by a vector has been shown to extend their natural host range. Similarly, inoculation of isolated protoplasts with virus can give rise to infection in cells of host species not known to be susceptible in nature. These findings suggest that the limiting factor with many plant viruses is their transmission and introduction into plant cells, rather than their capacity to exploit the host's biosynthetic machinery.

CAN PLANTS BE IMMUNIZED?

Active resistance systems bear a resemblance, albeit superficial, to the immune response of animals. This has led to repeated attempts to try to demonstrate the existence of a comparable immunological system in plants. To date, however, no post-infectional response involving the production of specific antibodies has been discovered in plants. Despite this negative result it has proved possible in a number of cases to immunize plants against virulent pathogens by employing techniques remarkably similar to those used in medicine.

Figure 9.5A diagrammatically represents a typical experiment. Prior inoculation of a leaf with an incompatible or heat-killed pathogen protects against infection by a live compatible pathogen administered several days later. This phenomenon has been demonstrated with numerous host-pathogen combinations and was instrumental in the discovery of phytoalexins. The conversion of a disease reaction type from susceptible to resistant by appropriate pretreatment has been variously termed acquired immunity, cross protection, interference and induced resistance. An obvious expla-

Table 9.2 Some types of induced resistance.

	TYPE	MECHANISMS	EXAMPLE	
			Pretreatment	Pathogen
Direct interactions	Antagonism	Antibiotics, bacteriocins, etc.	*Agrobacterium radiobacter*	*Agrobacterium tumefaciens*
	Occupation of penetration site	Mechanical obstruction	Rust fungi (block stomata)	Rust fungi
	Localized induced resistance	Phytoalexin accumulation	Incompatible race of *Phytophthora infestans*	Compatible race of *P. infestans*
Indirect interactions (host mediated)	Systemic induced resistance	Not known	*Colletotrichum lagenarium*	*Colletotrichum lagenarium*, tobacco mosaic virus and many other pathogens
	Viral cross protection	Not known	Avirulent tobacco mosaic virus	Virulent tobacco mosaic virus

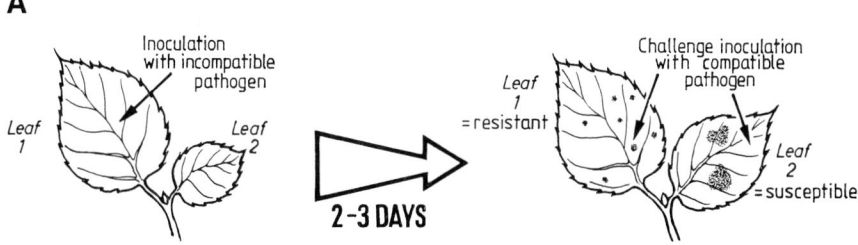

A

Inoculation
with incompatible
pathogen

Leaf 1   Leaf 2

2–3 DAYS

Challenge inoculation
with compatible
pathogen

Leaf 1 = resistant

Leaf 2 = susceptible

EXPERIMENTAL DEMONSTRATION OF LOCALIZED INDUCED RESISTANCE

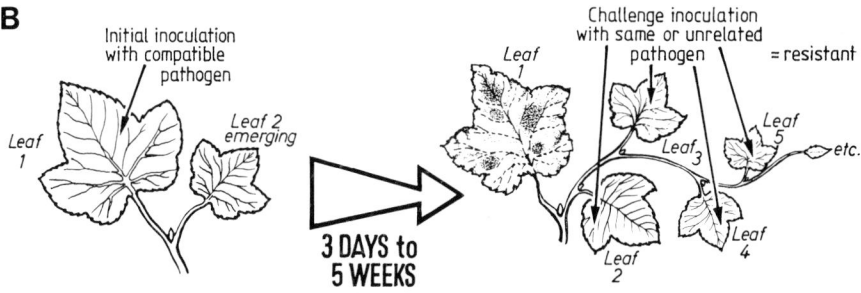

B

Initial inoculation
with compatible
pathogen

Leaf 2 emerging

Leaf 1

3 DAYS to 5 WEEKS

Challenge inoculation
with same or unrelated
pathogen = resistant

Leaf 1

Leaf 5

Leaf 3

etc.

Leaf 4

Leaf 2

EXPERIMENTAL DEMONSTRATION OF SYSTEMIC INDUCED RESISTANCE

Figure 9.5 Experimental sequences used to demonstrate the induction of disease resistance on a local or systemic basis.

nation for this diverse terminology is that several quite different mechanisms may be involved (Table 9.2). Some of these are simply due to direct interactions between the pretreatment and challenge inocula, while others are mediated by induced changes in the host.

The possibility of inducing resistance in plants raises intriguing prospects for disease control. However, many of these effects are ephemeral and localized, which obviously limits their value in agriculture. The likelihood that we can maintain an effective level of phytoalexin in a crop by continuously bombarding it with elicitors now seems naive. Nevertheless, at least some of the systems shown in Table 9.2 have found practical application in disease control. Direct interactions between microbes form the basis of several biological control methods discussed in Chapter 10. Systemic induced resistance (Fig. 9.5B) is a recent discovery most dramatically demonstrated in the family Cucurbitaceae. Treatment of the first leaf elicits systemic and long-lasting protection of all subsequently developing tissues. The protection is non-specific against various pathogens and effective under field conditions. The mechanism remains an enigma, and it is not known to what extent this type of induced resistance operates in other plant families.

Cross protection between viruses has no comparable counterpart in diseases caused by other pathogens. It only occurs between closely related viruses and various mechanisms, including formation of inhibitors and competition for essential building blocks, have been proposed to exploit the phenomenon. Cross protection has been exploited as a control method; for instance, protection of tomato plants against TMV by treatment with an attenuated strain of the same virus.

CONCLUSION

It is evident from this survey that plants have evolved a range of highly effective mechanisms to ward off microbial attack. Similarly, pathogens have evolved a variety of strategies for bypassing or suppressing these mechanisms. The fate of an invading organism is thus like that of a burglar who must pass through a series of doors to gain entry. Each door can either be open or locked but the intruder may be equipped with keys or other less subtle tools for breaking the doors down. To complicate matters, the first few doors in the sequence are linked by an alarm system to the later doors and tripping the alarm automatically activates the locks. There is, however, a delay in the system, and if the intruder moves quickly he can pass through all the doors before the locks engage. Finally, it should be remembered that the strength of the doors will not be the same in all cases. They may be damaged or defective or simply too old to function efficiently. Conversely, different intruders may possess differing degrees of strength and agility with which to force an entry!

FURTHER READING

General texts

DALY J.M. & URITANI I. eds (1979) *Recognition and Specificity in Plant Host-Parasite Interactions.* Japan Scientific Societies Press, Tokyo.
    A valuable collection of papers; see in particular contributions from Sequiera and Siegel.
DEVERALL B.J. (1977) *Defence Mechanisms of Plants.* Cambridge University Press, Cambridge.
    A standard text which explores many of the pertinent questions in physiological pathology.

Reviews and original articles

ALBERSHEIM P. & VALENT B.S. (1978) Host-pathogen interactions in plants. *Journal of Cell Biology* **78**, 627–43.
BUSHNELL W.R. & ROWELL J.B. (1981) Suppressors of defense reactions; A model for roles in specificity. *Phytopathology* **71**, 1012.
CALLOW J.A. (1977) Recognition, resistance, and the role of plant lectins in host-parasite interactions. *Advances in Botanical Research* **4**, 1–49.
DEVAY J.E. & ADLER H.E. (1976) Antigens common to hosts and parasites. *Annual Review of Microbiology* **30**, 147–68.
DIXON R.A. & LAMB C.J. (1980) The specificity of plant defences. *Nature* (London) **283**, 135–6.
DOKE N. & TOMIYAMA K. (1980) Suppression of the hypersensitive response of potato tuber protoplasts to hyphal wall components by water soluble glucans isolated from *Phytophthora infestans. Physiological Plant Pathology* **16**, 177–86.
HADWIGER L.A. & LOSCHKE D.C. (1981) Molecular communication in host-parasite interactions: hexosamine polymers (chitosan) as regulator compounds in race-specific and other interactions. *Phytopathology* **71**, 756–62.

KEEN N.T. (1981) Evaluation of the role of phytoalexins. In *Plant Disease Control* (eds Staples R.C. & Toenniessen G.H.), pp. 155–77. John Wiley & Sons, New York.

KUĆ J. (1981) Multiple mechanisms, reaction rates, and induced resistance in plants. In *Plant Disease Control* (eds Staples R.C. and Toenniessen G.H.), pp. 259–272. John Wiley & Sons, New York.

MOESTA P. & GRISEBACH H. (1980) Effects of biotic and abiotic elicitors on phytoalexin metabolism in soybean. *Nature* (London) **286**, 710–11.

WADE M. & ALBERSHEIM P. (1979) Race-specific molecules that protect soybeans from *Phytophthora megasperma* var. *sojae*. *Proceedings of the National Academy of Sciences, USA* **76**, 4433–7.

10 Disease control

"It was, finally, a matter of trying a large number of remedies, assuring myself of their merits, making them easy of execution, of taking into special account their economy of application, and of winning the confidence of the farmer."

M. TILLET (1714–1791)

Agriculture in many ways represents the antithesis of natural biological communities. The essential requirements for economically viable systems of crop husbandry are in basic conflict with most natural checks on pathogens. For example, monoculture of a single crop cultivar, manipulation of the environment through addition of fertilizers and climatic control within glasshouses all tend to favour those pathogens which can exploit the niches or situations so created. Hence, although disease remains the exception, the potential for explosive spread of the successful pathogen is enormously enhanced by comparison with natural communities.

Faced with this problem man has been forced to resort to any method of disease control which seems to offer a solution, albeit temporary.

In primitive agriculture, the predominantly small-scale operations included time-honoured rotations and other practices which tended to reduce disease losses. The demands of an ever-increasing world population have inevitably led to larger and more intensive agricultural regimes. At the same time the discovery of pesticides, many of which seemed to promise instant answers to the threat of disease, shifted attention to non-biological methods of control.

In the early part of this century, agricultural practice was further transformed by the application of genetic principles to plant breeding. This development led to improvements in the yield and quality of plant produce. Increased yield has been obtained by selection for both improved cropping and improved disease resistance. In addition, considerations of crop quality have become a major requirement of modern agriculture, and therefore influence the control measures adopted.

Unfortunately, the success of many of the control measures employed has been short-lived. The goal of a final solution to the problem of plant disease has remained illusory. The failure of chemists and plant breeders to provide permanent answers has recently refocussed attention on the application of ecological principles to disease control. Thus, the wheel has turned nearly full circle.

CHEMICALS AND DISEASE CONTROL

There is nowadays no shortage of critics eager to discredit the manufacturers and users of pesticides. This state of affairs has not, however, always been so and the excitement and relief which greeted the discovery of the first effective pesticides must have been similar to that generated by the introduction of penicillin. Today we are able to control pathogens and pests with a wide spectrum of chemicals suited to many different crop situations. The major exception to this concerns the viruses, which have so far defied all attempts at direct control by chemicals. There are several effective bacteriocides but we shall concentrate here on the fungicides and emphasize aspects of their development and deployment in agriculture.

The fascinating story of the early days of fungicide research has been ably recounted by E.C. Large in *The Advance of the Fungi*. We must now assess the current status of the science or, as some would have it, the art of chemical control of disease. The position has changed dramatically since the first fungicides, based on sulphur and copper, were discovered in 1846 and 1882 respectively. We now possess a wide spectrum of fungicidal compounds, these can be tailored to formulations which meet precise requirements, and we can apply the product with efficient machinery appropriate to a garden plot or a thousand hectare plantation.

Despite these advances one of the notable aspects of the modern fungicide scene is that if some of the pioneer plant pathologists, such as Berkeley or Millardet, were still alive today they would find in use several of the fungicides that they themselves had helped to develop (Fig. 10.1). Sulphur and copper are still the bases of recommended compounds with substantial sales. A similar longevity also seems to be assured for several of the organic fungicides discovered in the first half of this century. The dithiocarbamates, patented in 1934, and captan, which has been in use since 1949, are both still widely used. By contrast, some of the newer generations of compounds, while possessing remarkable properties as fungicides, have had to be withdrawn as they became biologically ineffective. It is ironic that this problem has arisen as in other respects the fungicide industry has succeeded in many of its major aims.

The perfect fungicide

It is relatively easy to construct a list of the desirable features one would like to see incorporated into a fungicide (Table 10.1). In practice, many problems are encountered in trying to achieve these aims. The biological considerations listed are attainable for many foliar and seed fungicides, but problems arise when the pathogen resides in the soil. Many soil fungicides have drastic results as they decimate the soil microflora and fauna. In fact, they are more correctly described as broad-spectrum biocides. Following their application the sterile soil will sooner or later be recolonized by a broad range of micro-organisms. Substantial benefits accrue if this col-

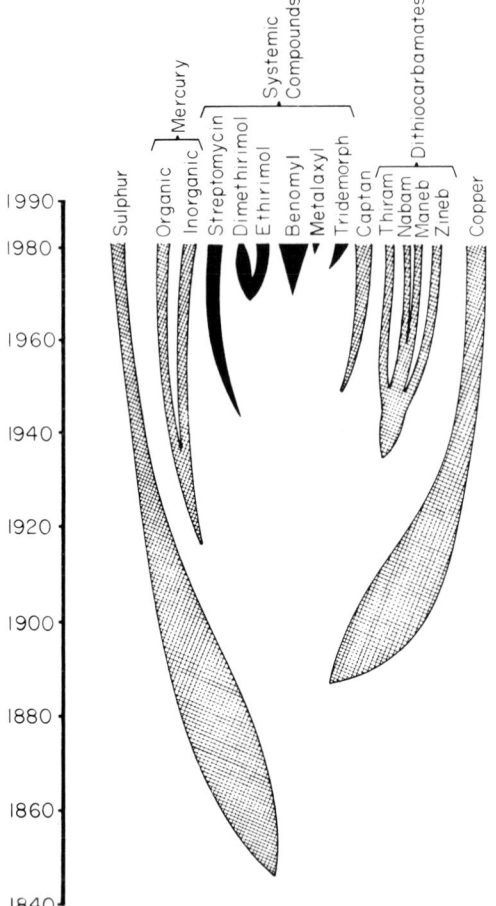

Figure 10.1 Evolution of fungicides; types available, origins and relative importance.

onizing microflora is dominated by fast-growing, nutritionally versatile saprophytes. Many such species are antagonistic to other organisms and hence their prior establishment in the soil will check the growth of any pathogen propagules which are re-introduced. *Trichoderma viride* is a fast-growing saphrophyte which is able to tolerate low levels of some biocides and is therefore an especially common recolonist following soil treatments with compounds such as chloropicrin and methyl bromide.

Following the introduction of systemic compounds, the persistence of fungicide residues in crops has posed an increasing problem. In some cases, however, materials are actually formulated to ensure their persistence, and they can thus be employed to reduce the incidence of damaging post-harvest diseases; this is certainly so with apples, citrus fruit and soft fruits. However, irrespective of the occurrence of post-harvest disease problems, the existence of such chemical residues must be seen as a potential threat to the consumer. Despite the existence of advisory and consumer-orientated organizations, too little attention seems to be paid to this problem. One

186

Table 10.1   Specifications of a perfect fungicide.

A. *Biological considerations*
    i. It must offer effective and consistent disease control.
    ii. It should not be phytotoxic at the recommended dose level.
    iii. It should not adversely affect other parts of the crop ecosystem.
B. *Toxicological considerations*
    i. It must not constitute a hazard during application.
    ii. Residues in the crop should not pose a problem for the consumer.
C. *Formulation factors*
    i. It should be safe to store and transport.
    ii. It should be simple to apply at a precise dosage level.
    iii. The method of formulation should increase its efficiency as a fungicide.
D. *Economic considerations*
    i. The financial return should exceed the cost of the fungicide and its application.

could perhaps envisage a "league table" for residue levels in fruits and vegetables, similar to that already published for the tar content of different cigarette brands!

Fungicide discovery and development

Many of the earlier generations of fungicides were discovered by accident or by the systematic examination of the properties of compounds which had originally been synthesized for other purposes. Thus copper was initially used to deter grape thieves and the dithiocarbamates were first developed as vulcanizing agents for the rubber industry. More recently, the quest for novel pesticides has come to involve teams of chemists and biologists who synthesize and test many thousands of compounds every year.

Regrettably, much of this endeavour remains empirical, with only vague guidelines being available to direct research. Although the research objectives are usually clear in terms of the potential market for new compounds, there is no guaranteed methodology for discovering chemicals with the desired biological activity. In addition, ever-higher hurdles have been erected to ensure that potential pesticides are both effective and safe. Thus, after the initial biological screening, there are now environmental and ecological screens through which compounds must pass if they are to be acceptable to the regulating authorities.

As a result of these stringent requirements, and the fact that new compounds must compete with the many effective pesticides already on the market, there has been a marked fall off in the rate at which commercially viable products have been discovered. For instance, in 1956 it was estimated that it was necessary to screen about 1800 compounds to find one new product, whereas in 1981 this ratio is now nearer to 15 000 : 1!

This dramatic decline in the agrochemical industry's success rate has considerable implications for the economics of pesticide development. The research costs involved add to the already huge budget needed to bring a compound into commercial use. Thus in 1981 it is estimated it will cost

£12 million to discover, develop and launch one new pesticide. This enormous sum must then be recouped in a relatively short time, as most patents cover a compound for only 20 years, and about half of that time will have been used up in the development and registration processes.

Protectant and systemic fungicides

Nearly all the fungicides discovered before 1960 came under the general description of PROTECTANT compounds (Table 10.2). These materials supplement the host's own defences by forming a superficial chemical barrier to prevent, or protect against, infection. Many effective protectant fungicides were discovered, but none of them was considered to be the perfect answer to the problem of disease control. By the very nature of their mode of action they must be applied before the pathogen attempts to penetrate the host. This emphasizes the need for reliable, early warnings of dispersal and the initiation of infection processes, if the materials are to be used effectively and economically. Because they form surface coatings protectant fungicides are subject to degradation and erosion by light, rain, and other environmental factors. Last, but not least, applications to growing plants rapidly become ineffective as leaves, flowers and fruits continue to develop.

In view of these disadvantages it is not surprising that a massive hunt went on for new types of fungicides. Chemists and biologists searched for SYSTEMIC compounds which could enter the host plant and, by operating from within, provide a semi-permanent addition to the plants own internal resistance mechanisms (Table 10.2). Systemic fungicides offer opportunities for therapy, i.e. the cure of an established infection, to be employed in combating disease. In this way plant pathology would become more like human medicine where the emphasis has always been on developing cures as well as preventing disease.

Table 10.2 Comparison of protectant and systemic fungicides.

	Protectant	Systemic
Action	Prophylactic	Therapeutic
Basis of toxicity	Many metabolic systems affected	Few metabolic systems affected
Phytotoxicity	Common, especially if applied to wrong tissue or an inappropriate host	Rare
Pathogens affected	Numerous	Variable – some extremely specific, others are effective against a broad spectrum
Pathogen resistance	Rare	Common
Movement	Confined to redistribution on surfaces	Translocated, usually in apoplast (xylem, cell walls)

One of the first compounds to be used as a systemic fungicide was the antibiotic streptomycin, but despite some successes, microbial metabolites have not proved to be very useful as fungicides. A number of exciting synthetic compounds have now been discovered which are taken up by plants and which are fungitoxic either directly or after they have been metabolized within the plant (Fig. 10.1). The movement of these materials through tissues obviates the need for accurate and widespread distribution over the host (Table 10.3). Unfortunately, most of these move only in the

Table 10.3 Effect of distribution on the efficiency of the protectant fungicide dinocap and the systemic fungicide benomyl on control of cucumber powdery mildew, *Sphaerotheca fuliginea*.

For each fungicide the same amount of material was applied per leaf in either one or a number of drops. After a period of incubation in an atmosphere laden with pathogen spores, the effects of the fungicides were assessed in terms of the area of leaf affected by the pathogen. The results are expressed as percentage reductions from control values. (After Evans, 1977.)

NO. DROPS PER LEAF	FUNGICIDE CONC PER DROP	DISEASE CONTROL (% reduction)	
		DINOCAP	BENOMYL
●	0·0250	5	20
● ●	0·0125	10	40
●● ●●	0·0067	20	100
●●●● ●●●●	0·0033	55	100
●●●● ●●●● ●●●● ●●●●	0·0017	100	100

apoplast and hence tend to travel from the seed or roots to the leaves and shoot apices; they do not circulate in the plant and in most tissues the effective concentration will thus decline unless there is continual uptake by the roots. This explains the success of seed dressing applications which can protect the plant for many weeks after germination—though the application of an expensive fungicide to the seed involves a measure of risk in the supposition that the subsequent disease levels will justify the treatment.

With the discovery of effective systemic fungicides it seemed for a while as if all the dreams of earlier years had come true. Disease after disease succumbed to these compounds, which can spread throughout the host and are not rapidly inactivated. However, problems have subsequently arisen in their use. Chief amongst these is the development of pathogens which can grow in the presence of high concentrations of fungicide.

Fungicide resistance

Prior to the discovery of the first systemic fungicides, there were very few occasions when protectant compounds failed to control a pathogen when applied at the correct time and at a previously established dosage level. Thus for decades the copper, sulphur and dithiocarbamate fungicides have remained as effective as when they were first discovered. The few exceptions to this rule include the remarkable case of *Pyrenophora avenae*, which managed to circumvent the drastic toxic effects of mercury applied as a seed dressing to oats. The regular use of diodine has resulted in the emergence of populations of the apple scab fungus (Fig. 10.2) able to withstand levels of this fungicide which were initially effective in controlling the disease. Similarly, the widespread use of diphenyl dips to prevent infection of citrus fruits by the post-harvest pathogen *Penicillium digitatum* led to changes in the fungus which enabled it to overcome the toxic effects of this compound. Despite the practical significance of these examples when they were discovered, they now seem unimportant in comparison with the situation which has developed since the introduction of systemic fungicides.

Changes in pathogen populations with respect to the effectiveness of fungicides are currently described in a number of ways. RESISTANCE is the preferred term for this phenomenon, but tolerance and insensitivity are also employed. Some authors prefer to use tolerance for instances where the change in the pathogen is due to a transient, physiological adaptation to the fungicide, rather than to a stable, genetic change, which is then described as resistance. However, as it is difficult in practice to distinguish between these two types of response, the two terms have come to be used interchangeably. It may, however, be argued that resistance is preferable, as tolerance does not convey the dramatic emphasis appropriate to a situation which has major biological and economic reverberations. Insensitivity is best kept to describe isolates of a pathogen at one end of the spectrum which occurs in any natural population, all members of which are effectively controlled by normal, recommended doses of the fungicide.

Acquired resistance to fungicides has now become an established fact of life in a world where systemic fungicides dominate large parts of the agricultural scene. An early example involved the pyrimidine fungicide dimethirimol. When this compound was introduced in 1968 it showed outstanding systemic activity against the cucumber powdery mildew pathogen, *Sphaerotheca fuliginea*. Initially, one soil drench containing 0.25 g of the compound protected plants for up to eight weeks, thus eliminating the previous routine of weekly spraying with a protectant compound. This product was taken up with great enthusiasm by the Dutch glasshouse industry but unfortunately the intensive use in that country quickly led to the emergence of highly resistant strains of the pathogen, and in 1971 the compound was withdrawn from use in the Netherlands. Thus a compound developed over many years was devalued after a tragically short lifespan.

Since that episode, there have been numerous other instances of

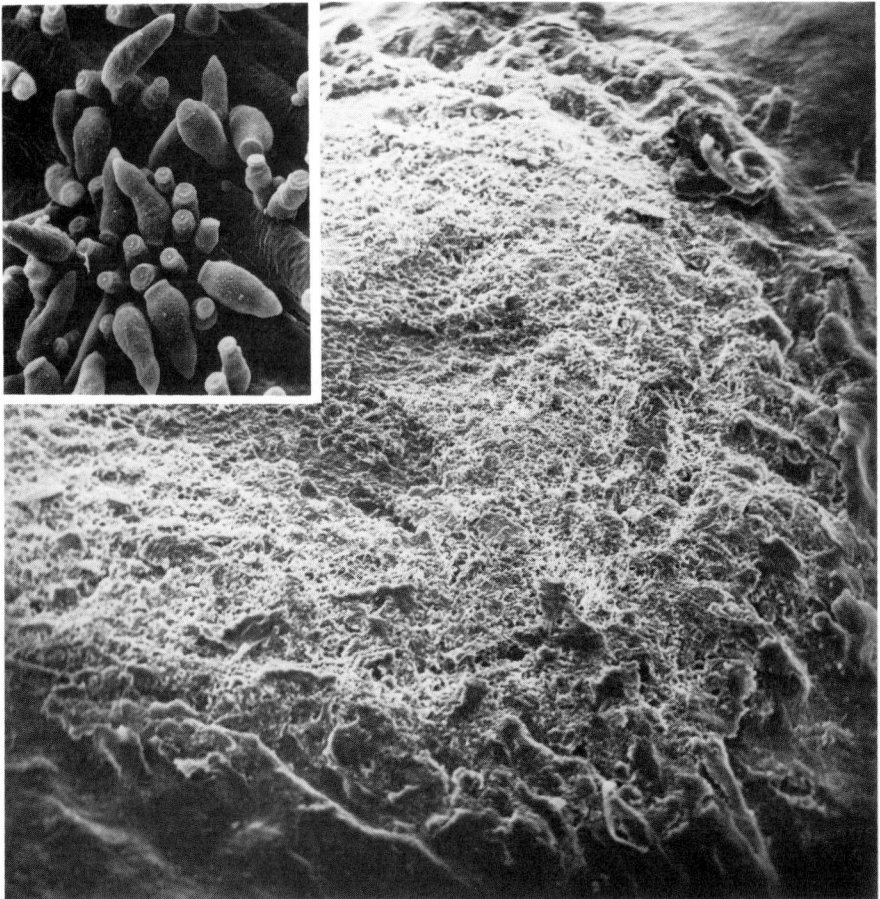

Figure 10.2   Scanning electron micrograph of a scab lesion on an apple fruit. Inset picture shows the pathogen's conidiophores emerging through the leaf cuticle and producing the elongate, two-celled, rain-dispersed conidia of *Venturia inaequalis*

fungicides becoming similarly ineffective. One of the most recent examples concerns the acylalanine fungicide metalaxyl, which aroused considerable interest when it was first released because of its ability to control phycomycetous fungi such as *Peronospora*, *Phytophthora* and *Pythium*. It also showed some ability to move in the symplast, an essential prerequisite for effective 'circulation' within the plant. Commercial formulations of this chemical, introduced in 1977–78, found ready application in many crops but unfortunately it was not long before the first signs of resistance emerged. In December 1979, isolates of *Pseudoperonospora cubensis* were found which were able to tolerate 20 times the level of fungicide needed to control sensitive isolates of this pathogen. More dramatically, in the following season there were instances of resistance occurring in populations of the potato blight pathogen, and this led to the manufacturers withdrawing those formulations which contained metalaxyl alone. Where metalaxyl has been formulated as a mixture with the dithiocarbamate mancozeb, it has remained effective and resistant strains have not become a problem. Its continued success when used in this way may be attributed to the presence of a powerful protectant material whose mode of action is very different from that of the metalaxyl.

Mode of action of fungicides

Most first-generation, protectant fungicides (see Fig. 10.1) are known to be MULTISITE pesticides, in that they interfere with the central metabolic processes of their victims. Indeed, the majority of these fungicides appear to affect the production of energy or ATP, either by inhibiting respiration or by uncoupling oxidative phosphorylation. Heavy-metal fungicides, such as cadmium and copper, inhibit a wide range of enzymes involved in various metabolic pathways. This fatal dislocation of the central core of the pathogen's metabolism probably explains why so few fungi have evolved systems enabling them to circumvent the toxic effects of these fungicides.

By contrast, a large number of the systemic compounds so far discovered operate at a SINGLE SITE in the cell, and hence resistance may arise as a consequence of mutation, which may involve only a single gene. Many of these compounds operate by disrupting the biosynthetic machinery of the cell, and hence deprive the fungus of supplies of new materials needed for growth. For example, the pyrimidines, e.g. dimethirimol and ethirimol, appear to be non-competitive inhibitors of enzymes involved in the biosynthesis of purines and amino acids, and the oxathiins, e.g. carboxin and oxycarboxin, prevent pathogen development by inhibiting succinate dehydrogenase. The widely used and versatile benzimidazoles, which include benomyl and thiabendazole, are transformed within the plant into highly active compounds which inhibit mitosis. A further group of systemic fungicides, including triarimol and triforine, inhibit sterol biosynthesis, while metalaxyl prevents the synthesis of RNA. Most of these systemic compounds are thus highly specific in their mode of action, and whilst this is in many ways desirable from an ecological and environmental viewpoint, it is their undoing as regards their continued effectiveness as fungicides.

A number of physiological and biochemical explanations have been advanced to explain the emergence of fungicide resistance. One obvious possibility is that the cell membranes of the pathogen become less permeable to the fungicide, so that insufficient enters the cells to build up a toxic concentration. If, however, the active compound does get inside the cell then it may be converted into non-toxic materials or alternatively the pathogen may cease to carry out a so-called lethal synthesis, whereby an initially non-toxic compound is metabolized into a highly toxic product. In other instances, the reactive site within the pathogen may show a decreased affinity for the fungicide; alternatively, if this site does become blocked then the pathogen may compensate for the loss of the usual biochemical reaction, either through a bypass mechanism or by enhanced activity elsewhere in the normal metabolic cycle.

Will resistance render all systemic compounds obsolete?

The history of the last two decades is not particularly auspicious when it comes to predicting the fate of the next generation of fungicides. Indeed, the problem of resistance, combined with the increasing difficulties involved in registration, must raise doubts as to whether there will be many more generations of fungicides! Fortunately, however, all is not lost and the lessons of recent years are being learnt, albeit rather late in the day.

Good fungicides, and for that matter good cultivars (see p. 202), must be carefully protected and conserved as an asset for the future. Hence a number of recommendations are emerging, which if followed will, we hope, stave off the possible development of resistance, or at worst minimize its importance (Table 10.4). It remains to be seen whether these measures will work, and whether they prove to be acceptable both to the agrochemical companies with an investment to recoup and to farmers with an urgent disease problem, which can seem like a matter of life or death at the height of an epidemic.

Table 10.4 Strategies designed to minimize the emergence of fungicide resistance (adapted from *Control of Diseases of Protected Crops and Cut Flowers*, ADAS Booklet 2364, HMSO, London).

1. Avoid repeated use of the same single-site fungicide or of materials with a similar mode of action.

2. When a programme of several sprays is needed in one season then:
   (a) whenever possible use manufacturer's formulations containing two or more fungicides
   (b) introduce multisite fungicides into the programme
   (c) reduce the number of sprays to the minimum by employing disease assessment, epidemiological and forecasting information.

3. Do not rely entirely on fungicides for disease control. Spray treatments should always be incorporated as part of a coordinated strategy, involving disease-resistant cultivars and cultural measures designed to minimize the spread of inoculum and pathogen.

Formulation and application

Formulation is the focus of much of the mystique attached to the agro-chemical industry. The tricks of how to get insoluble compounds into a suitable form for application, and then distribute them over a crop in such a way that they stick to plant surfaces and remain active for several days or even weeks, are closely guarded secrets. The discovery of systemic compounds has, to a certain extent, simplified the problems of formulation as once inside the plant these chemicals are no longer subject to the adverse effects of light and rain, which often result in the deterioration of materials residing on the surfaces of aerial plant tissues.

Numerous methods have been devised for applying fungicides to crops (Fig. 10.3), but in recent years several of these have come under scrutiny owing to the high energy costs involved. As before, the advent of systemic materials has somewhat eased the problem of application, in that accurate

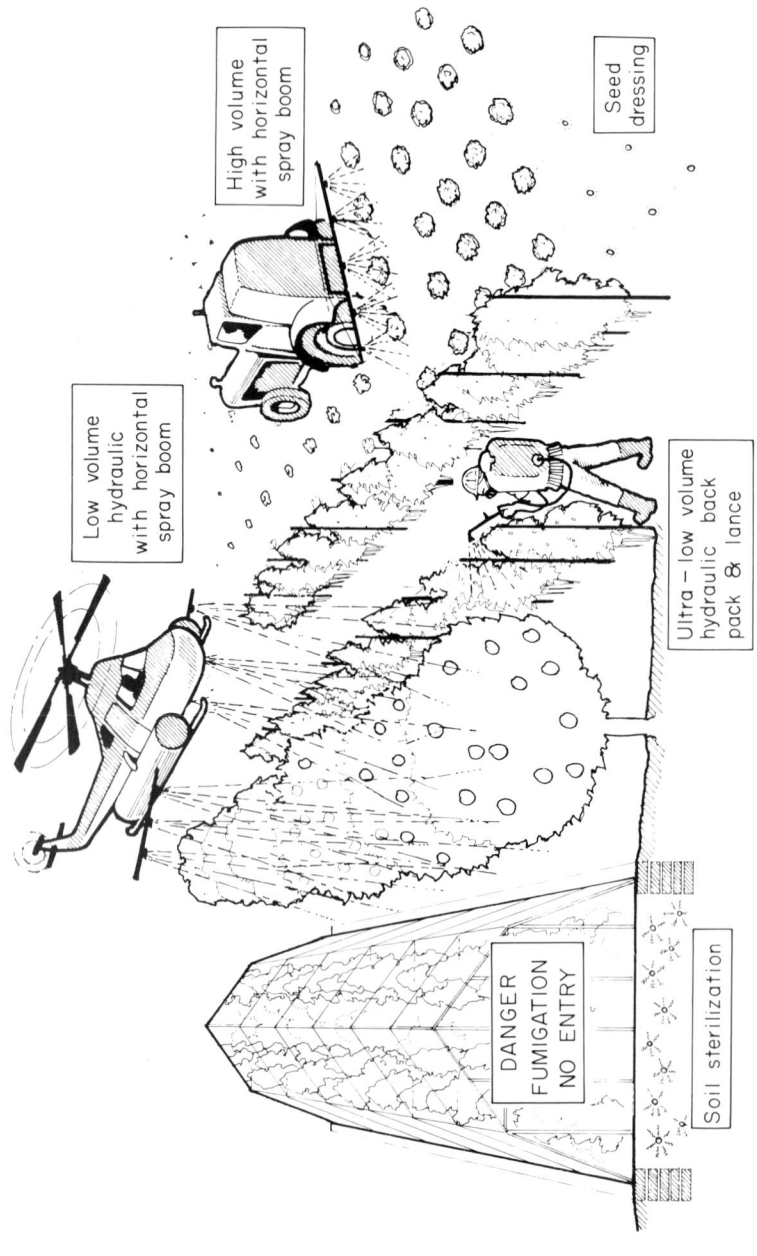

Figure 10.3 Some methods used to apply pesticides to various crops.

High volume with horizontal spray boom

Seed dressing

Low volume hydraulic with horizontal spray boom

Ultra – low volume hydraulic back pack & lance

DANGER FUMIGATION NO ENTRY

Soil sterilization

placement is now not always a high priority (Table 10.3). In addition, these fungicides have enabled progress to be made towards treating deep-seated pathogens, such as wilt fungi which inhabit the vascular system of plants. Dutch elm disease has been treated by injection of benzimidazole fungicides into the bole of elm trees but this method is expensive and the one-way movement of the fungicide quickly limits its efficacy. Future generations of systemics, which may move in the symplast as well as in the apoplast, should enable even greater progress to be made, with one major goal being the treatment of root-infecting pathogens, especially those affecting plantation crops.

Surface contaminants on seeds can be dealt with by simple dressings of powders or slurries. Protectant fungicides applied in this way only become active when the seed germinates, due to the availability of water. This ensures that the compound exerts its maximum effect when any pathogens are also resuming active growth. Deeper-seated infections can be treated with systemic compounds or, in a novel approach, by soaking seeds in solutions of protectant compounds, notably the dithiocarbamates. This technique depends upon careful timing of the soak to avoid germination commencing, and the seed is then dried and sown in the normal way. The treatment is only economically viable for small, relatively-valuable seeds such as those of celery and cauliflower.

Whither pesticides?

The economics of chemical disease control are, in theory, simple. Weigh up the disease losses and the total cost of the control measure and see if a profit is indicated. In practice, as was discussed in Chapter 3, the main problem lies in the first part of the equation. Disease losses can only be forecast, often with a very limited degree of accuracy. Even using elaborate computer predictions, serious discrepancies have occurred between predicted and actual amounts of disease. Only when we have reliable models which enable us to make accurate forecasts will chemical control measures be used most economically and with minimum risk to the consumer and the environment.

Despite the counter attractions of other forms of disease control there is no doubt as to the benefits which accrue from the use of chemicals on a country-wide scale. For instance, it has been calculated that if pesticides were banned in the USA, agricultural output would fall by up to 30%, resulting in price increases of 50–75%.

Most attention has been directed here towards fungicides, as the state of the art is far more advanced than it is for bacteriocides or viricides. Bacteria have been mainly controlled by copper compounds and the antibiotic streptomycin. The former are still effective but arouse great suspicion amongst ecologists, whereas the latter has become less effective in recent years owing to the emergence of resistant strains of bacteria. As the use of further antibiotics, especially those employed in human medicine, is considered undesirable, it is imperative that we discover new bacteriocides, preferably with systemic properties. Such materials would find a ready market in many countries but particularly in the tropics, where there are many major bacterial pathogens affecting rice, citrus, cucurbits and other crops.

No antiviral agents effective against plant-pathogenic viruses have yet been discovered. Indeed, the study of such materials is still in its infancy even in the more intensively studied field of animal pathology. It has nevertheless been shown that symptoms due to plant viruses can be alleviated by certain chemicals, including the fungicide carbendazim, and this suggests that there may be exciting developments in this area in the not-too-distant future.

In all the examples given in this section the emphasis has been on chemicals which have a direct toxic effect on a target micro-organism. When considering the long-term future of chemical control of disease it may be appropriate to conclude by mentioning some chemicals which have been termed antipathogenic. These compounds, which have little toxicity towards the pathogen *in vitro*, prevent the establishment of an effective parasitic relationship. Whether they do so by 'turning on' the plant's own defence mechanisms or by interfering with the enzymes involved in the establishment of the parasitic relationship is not known, but clearly their development may prove to be the next landmark in the long history of the chemical control of plant disease.

BREEDING FOR RESISTANCE

In many ways, plant breeding may be regarded as a form of biological control, but as its application involves an array of distinct techniques and broad economic considerations, it will be discussed here under a separate heading.

The introduction of crop cultivars containing new genes is a normal ingredient of modern agriculture and, apart from the arguments surrounding genetic uniformity (see below), the process does not have serious environmental consequences. Indeed, at one time breeding for resistance seemed to promise an ideal and permanent solution to the problem of plant disease.

Up until the end of the nineteenth century, plant breeding was essentially empirical. In spite of this it must have played an important part in restricting disease losses. In years when disease epidemics wiped out most of the crop, it automatically followed that only the most resistant plants survived to provide seed for the following season. This sequence was merely an extension of the process of natural selection which maintains an equilibrium between a pathogen and its host in natural communities. At the same time the gradual development of the intuitive art of breeding, whereby higher-yielding and more resilient individuals were progressively selected, undoubtedly included an element of selection for resistance to disease.

The foundations of the scientific process of breeding for disease resistance were laid by Biffen early this century. By 1912 he had shown that resistance to yellow stripe rust in the wheat cultivar Rivet was determined by a single recessive gene the inheritance of which obeyed Mendel's laws. This discovery triggered off a massive programme aimed at introducing similar resistance into other important crops. At first it seemed all too easy; all that was apparently required was the introduction into a crop of a suitable gene for resistance which was then built in as a permanent feature. What had not been anticipated, however, was that the pathogen was also capable of conducting its own breeding programme! The introduction of a new host gene for resistance was regularly followed by the appearance of a new race of the pathogen capable of overcoming the effects of this gene. This in turn led to a renewed search for resistance genes which were again frequently countered by changes in the pathogen. An example of this type of sequential introduction of genes is seen in the development of barley cultivars resistant to powdery mildew (Fig. 10.4). Resistance genes from a variety of sources were countered with monotonous regularity.

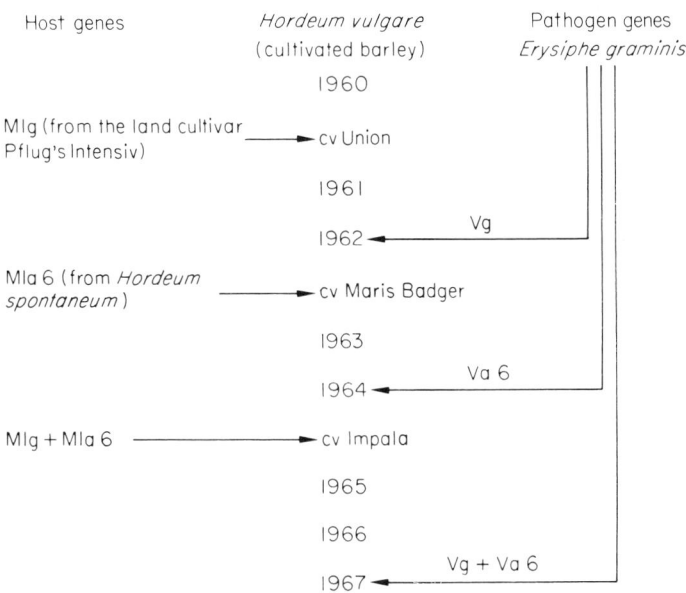

Figure 10.4 Successive introductions into the United Kingdom barley crop of cultivars containing genes for resistance to powdery mildew and the subsequent selection for virulence genes in the *Erysiphe* population.

The boom-and-bust cycle

The rate at which the pathogen responds to newly created selection pressures depends upon several factors. Foremost amongst these is the proportion of the total crop area given over to the novel cultivar (Fig. 10.5). The widespread planting of a particular cultivar containing one or a few resistance genes will inevitably favour pathogen races containing the

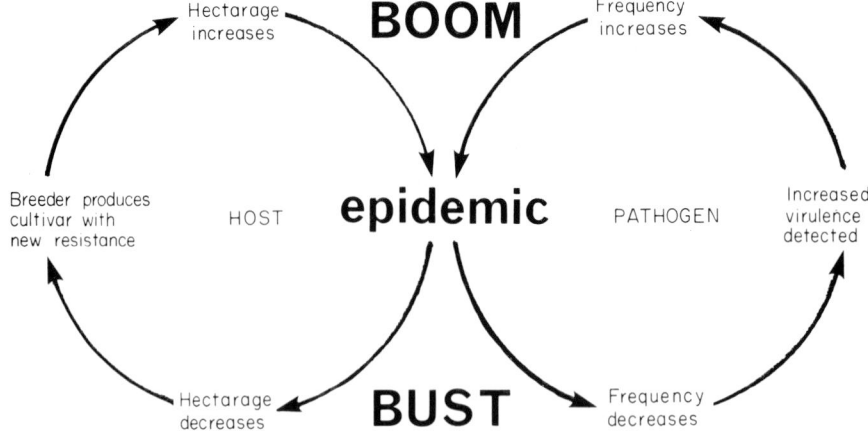

Figure 10.5   The boom-and-bust cycle (from Priestley, 1978).

appropriate virulence genes, a process known as directional selection. For example, the popularity of the barley cultivar Sultan was thought to be largely responsible for the rapid rise in the level of virulence towards this cultivar within the *Erysiphe graminis* population (Table 10.5). This shift in the make-up of the pathogen population then quickly resulted in a decline in the area planted with Sultan. Other factors influencing the dynamic changes in the host–pathogen balance include the pre-existing frequency of occurrence of virulence to any new cultivar, the level of this virulence and the ability of virulent strains to flourish on both non-resistant and relatively resistant cultivars.

This game of 'cat and mouse' has continued to the present day, with only a few exceptions in the form of genes which have remained effective against a particular pathogen for more than a few years. For instance, resistance of potato to *Synchytrium endobioticum* has remained effective for over 50 years and some wheat cultivars have had a long-lasting resistance to eyespot caused by *Pseudocercosporella herpotrichoides*. In the former example, the resistance genes have been protected to a certain extent by regulations which forbid the planting of potatoes in soils known to be infested with the pathogen. Eyespot is, however, a prevalent disease and the failure of *Pseudocercosporella* to overcome the resistance which has been introduced

Table 10.5   History in the United Kingdom of the barley cultivar Sultan with respect to its resistance to naturally occurring races of *Erysiphe graminis*.

	1967	1968	1969	1970	1972
Area planted (% of whole area of spring barley)	<1	9	21	30	6
Erysiphe infection index (Mean of all cultivars grown = 100)	34	43	32	123	189
Pathogen virulence	First seen	Rare	Common	Very common	Very common

makes this a good example of long-lasting success achieved by plant breeding.

A partial answer to the problem posed by new races of pathogens is to foretell their appearance and then act quickly to phase out non-resistant cultivars. Pathologists now periodically sample pathogen populations which occur naturally in growing areas and determine the spectrum of races present. They can also use laboratory experiments to speed up the processes thought to be occurring in nature. Such information cannot be used to prevent the new races from appearing but it can allow growers to switch to resistant cultivars and so avoid catastrophic losses.

An alternative strategy is to deploy individual resistance genes in a more carefully regulated and diversified manner, thereby stabilizing the selection of any particular virulence genes in the pathogen population (see below).

The breeder's treadmill

The current situation in which new cultivars are quickly rendered obsolete by new races of the pathogen has been to a large extent a legacy of breeding for oligogenic types of resistance (see Chapter 3). This trend is predictable inasmuch as oligogenic resistance is readily identified and, being based upon very few genes, it can easily be manipulated in a breeding programme (Table 10.6). Its great disadvantage lies in its specificity towards only one or a few races of the pathogen. Thus there is a high chance of a new race being able to overcome its effects. This hard-earned lesson has led to increased interest in polygenic types of resistance, based upon many genes.

Unfortunately it is difficult to study this form of resistance due to the lack of clear-cut disease-reaction types. It has even been argued that such

Table 10.6 Main points of contrast between oligogenic and polygenic resistance (from Hayes & Johnston, 1971).

	Oligogenic	Polygenic
Genetic control	Few genes involved	Usually many genes involved
Description	Generally clear cut; functions throughout life of plant, or may be expressed in mature plants only	Variable; seedlings generally less resistant, but resistance increases as plants mature
Mechanism	Generally a hypersensitive host reaction	Reduced rate and degree of infection, development and/or reproduction of pathogen
Efficiency	Highly efficient, but often extremely low resistance to other races	Variable, effective against all races of pathogen
Stability	Liable to suddenly break down due to the development of new physiologic races of the pathogen	Not affected by changes in virulence genes of the pathogen
Commonly used approximate synonyms	Vertical Major gene Seedling Race-specific	Horizontal Minor gene Adult plant Race-non-specific Field

resistance is a purely theoretical concept and impossible to substantiate, as a pathogen must be shown to be incapable of evolving increased virulence which would enable it to overcome that resistance. In practice, however, there are cultivars which exhibit susceptible responses in greenhouse or growth-room tests but are nevertheless relatively resistant in the field, and these cultivars have been described as possessing polygenic resistance.

A more concrete concept, which has immense practical value, is that of DURABLE resistance. This type of resistance cannot be attributed to any particular mechanism or genetic model and the only reliable criterion for its recognition is that it remains effective over long periods in the field. Examples include the aforementioned resistance to eyespot, which in the wheat cultivar Cappelle-Desprez has remained effective for more than 20 years, and the resistance to yellow stripe rust shown by a number of wheat cultivars. A more dramatic example is provided by certain barley cultivars which avoid infection by the loose smut fungus, *Ustilago nuda*, because their flowers do not open and hence the stigmata, through which the fungus enters the host, are physically protected.

It is tempting to equate durable resistance with polygenic resistance but there is little evidence to support such a conclusion. In practical terms, polygenic resistance remains something of an enigma, but durable resistance is an observed fact and breeding schemes have been devised to search for further examples of this valuable characteristic.

Production of novel disease-resistant plants

Can the breeding of new resistant crop cultivars continue indefinitely? To answer this question we must consider the sources of the most important ingredient in the process, namely the germ plasm which confers resistance. We also need to ask how this resistance may be combined with other agronomically desirable traits to produce new cultivars.

Traditionally, resistance genes have been sought either within a crop species or in wild relatives. In the early days of plant breeding, crop species exhibited considerable variation, and selection from within the existing population could produce major shifts in the crop's level of resistance. This approach remains of value with many crops, especially when screening for previously unsought types of resistance, such as adult plant resistance which cannot be detected in seedlings. Where domesticated crop species themselves have failed to yield any effective sources of resistance, attention has shifted to their wild relatives.

If the relationship between such wild species and the crop concerned is sufficiently close, then hybridization by conventional means is usually a comparatively simple process. For instance, wild relatives of the potato, tomato and tobacco have been successfully used as sources of genes conferring resistance against late blight, leaf mould and TMV respectively. In other instances, it has proved impossible to cross potentially useful plants and hence novel techniques for the creation of interspecific and intergeneric hybrids are now being developed. These methods aim to bypass the natural compatibility barriers which normally preclude such hybridization. Advances in this area have to a large extent depended upon developments in plant tissue culture, whereby organs, single cells or protoplasts can be manipulated *in vitro* and then regenerated into intact plants. Certain compatibility barriers operating after fertilization can, for instance, be overcome by removing the young embryo and nursing it to maturity under sterile conditions. In other cases where sexual hybrids have proved impossible to obtain, the fusion of somatic (i.e. vegetative) cells may eventually provide a reliable technique for introducing resistance genes into crops from entirely unrelated plant species.

An alternative approach is to introduce specific genes into plant cells utilizing transformation techniques based upon recombinant-DNA technology. One, perhaps ironic, aspect of this approach is that a bacterial plant pathogen, *Agrobacterium tumefaciens*, may itself prove useful as a means of introducing new genetic information into plant cells by virtue of its Ti plasmid (see Chapter 8). The wide host range of this bacterium, coupled with the fact that part of the plasmid is actually incorporated into the host cell nucleus and becomes stably expressed, suggests that it may be an ideal vehicle for inserting foreign DNA into a plant genome. While the possibilities offered by these methods appear endless, it should be noted that major problems in the identification and isolation of the necessary resistance genes have still to be solved; also, it remains to be seen whether transferred genes will be effectively expressed in a recipient host cell. As we saw in previous chapters, resistance comprises a number of components. Thus the notion that the transfer of a single gene specifying, for example, phytoalexin synthesis might convert a susceptible plant into a resistant one, while attractive in its simplicity, seems unlikely to work in practice.

Whatever method is employed to introduce genes into a crop, there is a limit to the world's stock of such genes, and the continual development of new cultivars must eventually exhaust the supply. We would then be forced to rely upon induced mutations to create a supply of novel germ plasm. Attempts have already been made to produce useful mutants, but owing to our incomplete knowledge of the existing spectrum of genes, it is difficult to determine whether these have resulted in the creation of any unique genes. To be effective, mutation methods require large-scale experiments in which huge numbers of plants can be screened. Here again, tissue culture may assist us by allowing screening of cells rather than whole plants, thus facilitating detection of mutations which occur at very low frequencies. A further possibility is to try to select for resistant cells utilizing a pathogen-produced toxin as the selection agent. In diseases where a host-specific toxin is involved, this type of strategy has already proved feasible. Resistant cells which survive exposure to toxin can then be regenerated to give resistant plants. The advantages over conventional techniques in terms of both numbers of individuals processed and the time involved are obvious.

Recent experiments in which protoplasts isolated from the leaves of certain potato cultivars were regenerated to give clones of new plants have shown that novel morphological variants can be recovered by this process. The mechanism underlying such variation is not entirely clear, although one explanation is that in the original leaf tissues the individual cells form a 'genetic mosaic'. The important implication from a pathological point of view is that similar variations may extend to disease resistance. More work is needed to assess whether this phenomenon applies to other crop species. If, however, cloning from isolated cells or protoplasts should reveal hitherto undiscovered variation in long-established crop cultivars, then attempts to introduce exotic genes from distant species may be unnecessary! Instead, breeders will be able to concentrate on the more traditional approach of selecting the resistant individuals from within a population.

Deployment of genetic resistance in the field

In the past no attempt was made to coordinate or conserve genetic resources. Seedmerchants promoted, and farmers planted, a sequence of cultivars, each of which represented an improvement on the last in terms of yield, which in every instance would have been contributed to by factors conferring resistance to disease. The effective commercial life of cultivars was determined by their continued success in large-scale agriculture and by the introduction of further cultivars which offered the promise of even higher yields.

In recent years it has become apparent that this *ad hoc* system does not allow for an orderly and efficient use of the world's stock of genetic resources. Indeed, it has been pointed out that we have frequently squandered valuable resistance genes in order to achieve short-term gains, to the point where in some crops there are few, if any, novel genes left to be deployed. Hopefully, this chaotic state of affairs is coming to an end. Various trade and governmental bodies are now attempting to promote schemes designed to prolong the usefulness of cultivars by making it more difficult for virulent strains of the pathogen to flourish (Table 10.7). The procedures listed in this table are not necessarily applicable to each and every disease, and indeed in some instances there are few, if any, known sources of resistance to particular pathogens.

The common theme in these different strategies is diversification, thereby avoiding simultaneous exposure of a single resistance gene over a wide area. However, fears have been expressed that such genetic diversification could conceivably favour the emergence of pathogen super-races virulent towards numerous host resistance genes.

Future trends in plant breeding for disease resistance

Experience to date suggests that airborne pathogens would be most effectively controlled by the introduction of polygenic resistance into crops, whereas soil-borne pathogens, which generally cause less explosive epide-

Table 10.7 Deployment of resistance genes to ensure their maximum continued effectiveness.

A. Action by plant breeders
1. To develop multigene cultivars, in which more than one resistance gene is combined in a single cultivar.
2. To develop multiline cultivars, made up of a series of cultivars identical in agronomic characters but differing in specific resistance genes.
B. Action by seedmerchants
1. To market mixtures of cultivars with different agronomic characters including a different genetic basis for their resistance.
C. Action by pathologists and farmers
1. To encourage the restricted use of resistance genes, e.g. by using them in defined geographical areas or in only one of a number of overlapping cropping systems, such as either winter or spring sown cereals.
2. To encourage farmers to adopt diversification schemes whereby they grow a different cultivar in each of their fields. These are selected from groups of cultivars known to have a different genetic basis for disease resistance.

mics, might be effectively dealt with by the use of oligogenic resistance. Some progress has been made towards this goal and for a few diseases, which are regarded as highly important, there is an enormous amount of genetic information available, together with a wide range of well-characterized resistance genes. By contrast, for other diseases, and indeed for some crops, there is a lamentable lack of knowledge and this state of affairs is not likely to be rectified in the near future.

This uneven situation is a product of the climate in which breeding for disease resistance is carried out. Commercial plant breeders must develop cultivars which farmers will want to grow. Only then will sufficient royalties be generated to fund future breeding programmes. In deciding their breeding strategy, the question of disease resistance is only one of many to be considered. Indeed, in some cases there is doubt as to the priority which farmers place on high levels of disease resistance, especially since the advent of the highly successful systemic fungicides. As fungicides become more expensive and less acceptable to consumers, however, this situation will alter, placing a renewed emphasis on plant breeding as a means of disease control.

Despite the many past failures and disappointments, plant breeding still has a vital contribution to make to disease control. Several new approaches are being developed, and a conspicuous effort is being made to reverse the trends of the past century by increasing the amount of genetic variation in crops. This major reappraisal was precipitated to some extent by the 1970 epidemic of southern corn leaf blight in the USA. What had been hailed as a breakthrough in breeding techniques became a hazard, as the male sterility factor concerned was found to be linked to susceptibility towards *Helminthosporium* blight. This disastrous epidemic removed much of the gloss from modern plant breeding. As a result, many other important crops, including dwarf wheat, rice, sorghum and sugar beet, came under scrutiny and all were found to possess a very narrow genetic base, especially where disease resistance was concerned. As already discussed, the tendency for one or a few closely related cultivars to come to predominate over wide areas added to this uniformity and increased the likelihood of large-scale disease epidemics occurring. One hopes that such problems will soon be forgotten as the positive aspects of plant breeding are developed within the framework of an integrated approach to plant disease control.

BIOLOGICAL CONTROL

Microbial pathogens growing within host tissues are not usually subject to interference by other micro-organisms. However, during dispersal, survival and the early stages of infection, pathogens are vulnerable to attack by free-living organisms. Plant pathologists have belatedly come to recognize the potential of this natural antagonism towards pathogens, and to exploit it in the process known as BIOLOGICAL CONTROL.

Biological control is not a new concept; indeed it has been practised for as long as chemical control. However, until relatively recently almost all the spectacular successes in this field involved pests or weeds.

The first biological control system to be used on a field basis involved the cotton-cushion scale insect. This pest was first recorded in California in 1868 and it subsequently spread rapidly through the newly established citrus groves. Entomologists suspected that the pest had come from Australia, probably on imported nursery stock, and a search was made there for natural predators. Two of these, a lady beetle and a fly, were selected for trials. These were imported and released in California in 1888 and within a few months the problem of cotton-cushion scale had been solved.

The principle involved in this example is devastatingly simple and yet extremely effective. Pests are almost certain to have natural enemies somewhere in the world and these are introduced to reduce the offending populations. Of course, there have been failures, particularly as introduced species have not always become successfully established in their new habitats. However, this approach has remained viable to the present day and over 100 examples can be cited to testify to its success.

Amongst these examples are several involving introduced plants which have become serious weeds. The most infamous case of such a weed was the prickly pear cactus, *Opuntia*, which was introduced into Australia as a hedging plant. Unfortunately it prospered so well in that country that it colonized and ruined enormous areas of valuable pasture before its spread was halted by caterpillars and mealy bugs brought from its native South America.

One potential hazard of introducing any species into a new area is that it may be difficult to foresee all the eventual ecological consequences. This caution applies especially to introduced predators and pests. The herbivorous beetles introduced into North America and Australia to control Klamath weed (*Hypericum perforatum*) were carefully selected to avoid species which might have turned their attention to useful forage plants once the weed had been controlled.

The success of these biological control systems may be ascribed to a number of factors. By virtue of their size, pests and weeds are more easily studied than are micro-organisms. The occurrence and effects of predators are, therefore, easily monitored. Quite apart from these methodological advantages there would also seem to be some fundamental features of pest–predator systems which man can exploit. In every ecosystem there is a remarkable variety of invertebrates occupying all trophic levels. Many species have a limited geographic distribution. In contrast, there are probably fewer species of fungi and bacteria and many of these have a cosmopolitan distribution. Hence there is less chance of finding specific antagonists of microbial pathogens, either locally or in other continents. Even where such antagonists are discovered, the interactions between them and the pathogen are often less dramatic than amongst invertebrates, where predators normally kill their victims outright.

These comparisons assume that a microbial pathogen will probably be antagonized by another micro-organism, while invertebrates are attacked only by other invertebrates. This is the more usual situation, but there are some intriguing instances where micro-organisms parasitize invertebrates. A number of soil fungi are known to enjoy a diet of nematodes, which they trap or capture by various mechanisms. As yet it has not been possible to exploit this discovery, probably because of our lack of knowledge of the environmental factors which favour these nematophagous fungi. Other fungi, such as *Beauvaria* and *Metarrhizium*, parasitize insects. Development of these as agents of biological control has got as far as pilot industrial plants for the production of fungal inocula to be sprayed on crops affected by insect pests. Bacteria and viruses are also being used to control insects and both *Bacillus thuringiensis* and the baculo viruses appear to be promising in this respect.

Introduction of specific antagonists

To date, there have been relatively few successful schemes for the biological control of microbial plant pathogens. In particular, there are few instances where the principle of introducing a specific antagonist has been employed. This is, to a large extent, due to the common experience that the introduced species fails to flourish in the desired manner. This failure may be explained by the general ecological maxim that the constitution of a community occupying a habitat reflects the nutritional and environmental conditions in that habitat and that if the antagonist could succeed it would have done so already. Hence, the introduction of a single species into a complex community, such as is found on the leaf surface or in soil, is almost certainly doomed to failure.

There are, however, apparent exceptions to this rule; if these are examined more closely it will often be seen that the introduction of the antagonist has been accompanied by an alteration in the ecosystem, ranging from the prior application of a biocide, to a dramatic increase in the population of the pathogen itself. Under these circumstances there may be more chance that the introduced antagonist will successfully become established.

An excellent illustration of this concept is provided by the scheme devised to control *Heterobasidion annosum*, which causes heart rot of pines. Air borne basidiospores of this fungus colonize stump surfaces of newly felled trees. The mycelium then spreads to adjacent living trees by growing along the root systems. Chemical control measures only delay infection, as the concentration of fungicide in the stump eventually declines to a point where *Heterobasidion* can become established. A perfect solution to the problem was devised in 1963 when Rishbeth inoculated cut stumps with *Peniophora*, a wood-rotting parasite/saphrophyte which is antagonistic to *Heterobasidion*. Commercially produced spore suspensions are now used to paint the stump surfaces immediately after felling, or they can even be added to the lubricating oil used on the chain saw. Satisfactory control is regularly achieved. It must be appreciated that this example involves somewhat unusual conditions, in that the newly exposed surface of the stump presents a virgin substrate for microbial colonization, and hence the antagonist does not face any great problems in establishing itself.

A further, somewhat comparable, example of a biological control measure which is dependent upon the *de novo* creation of a sterile infection court is that used for apple canker. The pathogen, *Nectria galligena*, regularly enters its host via the abscission scars which are left when apple leaves are shed in autumn. When the leaves fall, these scars are only partially sealed off and the vascular elements form natural openings through which this pathogen may enter the woody branch. Extensive systematic investigations showed that other organisms also colonize these openings and when one of these, the bacterium *Bacillus subtilis*, was present it prevented the apple canker pathogen from becoming established. This discovery has been exploited by applying a spray treatment shortly after leaf fall consisting of a suspension of bacterial cells.

Both the above systems of biological control depend for their success upon interactions in a specific infection court. Other examples can be found which follow this theme, but there is one outstanding biological control scheme for which there is no such requirement. This concerns the control of crown gall disease caused by *Agrobacterium tumefaciens*. A closely related species, *Agrobacterium radiobacter*, has been successfully used to control this disease in many parts of the world. One strain of this saprophytic bacterium is remarkably active in inhibiting infection when applied to seeds, cuttings, graft unions or bare roots. This antagonism appears to be due to the production of an extracellular toxin, known as a bacteriocin, which inactivates the pathogen. Not all isolates of the pathogen are equally sensitive to this strain of *A. radiobacter* and a further search is needed to find other successful antagonists.

It is remarkable that *A. radiobacter* is effective in so many situations and it highlights our failure to find comparable systems for other microbial pathogens. Despite this, the spectacular achievements of the currently effective schemes have encouraged plant pathologists to take a renewed interest in biological control.

Manipulation of natural populations

Many other examples of biological control of microbial plant pathogens involve manipulation of the environment to stimulate selectively naturally occurring control processes. We have already seen that many plant pathogens spend part of their life cycle in soil. Here they are subject to competition from the rest of the soil microflora. It is possible to manipulate the soil ecosystem in a variety of ways to the disadvantage of the pathogen, and these processes constitute a form of biological control.

It has been known for a very long time that crop rotation is an important factor in the control of many diseases. Populations of the take-all pathogen can be substantially reduced by a two- to three-year rotation to grass leys. The eradication of *Gaeumannomyces* has been shown to result from the build-up of the population of an antagonistic fungus, *Phialophora radicicola*, which is especially common on the surfaces of grass roots. Green manure has also been used to alter soil conditions in favour of harmless saphrophytes. Potato scab has been controlled in this way, by alternating potatoes with soybeans, which are ploughed in while still green prior to planting the main crop. The control which is achieved is thought to be due to the selective encouragement of *Bacillus subtilis* which is antagonistic to *Streptomyces scabies*.

Other types of nutrient amendment have been employed in disease control. The apple scab pathogen overwinters as a stroma in infected leaves and fruits lying on the orchard floor. Re-infection of newly expanding leaves in spring is by ascospores released from ascocarps which have developed within these stromata. The addition of nitrogen, in the form of urea, to newly fallen leaf litter ensures that the non-parasitized tissues are quickly destroyed by saprophytes. This results in fewer ascocarps being formed in the following spring, probably because the pathogen is unable to obtain nutrients from beyond the margin of the stroma.

More recently it has been recognized that pathogen–saprophyte interactions are not confined to the soil environment. The idea that biological control operated on aerial tissues was suggested as long ago as 1910 by Potter, who demonstrated that viable non-pathogenic microbes were present on leaf surfaces. Many years passed before serious attention was given to the practical implications of his suggestion. Antagonism occurs on aerial plant surfaces, though it is probably less common in these habitats than in the soil. The surfaces of stems, leaves, flowers and fruits are often inhospitable for micro-organisms, but favourable conditions for growth occur in the humid tropics or, in temperate regions, within dense crop canopies. Opportunities for antagonism also exist because many microbes have adapted to the fluctuating, and often extreme, environments which are characteristic of these exposed plant organs. After all, if pathogens are able to grow across these surfaces to locate suitable infection sites it is hardly surprising that saprophytes are also able to flourish in the same environment.

The knowledge that interactions can occur on aerial plant surfaces does not, however, tell us how important they are or how they may be manipulated in a useful manner. Both questions remain largely unanswered. There is circumstantial evidence suggesting that naturally occurring biological control has been grossly underestimated but proof of this is still relatively sparse. For example, it is known that *Tuberculina maxima* is a common inhabitant of the cankers caused by the rust *Cronartium ribicola* on *Pinus*. There is evidence that *Tuberculina* can reduce the inoculum potential of the rust by competing for or destroying its food source in the pine. Hence it would seem likely that it can act as a useful natural check on the rust, but definite proof of its importance is not yet forthcoming. The question of how we may manipulate microbial populations on leaves and stems raises even more interesting problems and possibilities, but so far no convincing schemes have been developed.

Mechanisms involved in microbial antagonism

A list of the mechanisms of antagonism between micro-organisms is given in Table 10.8. Several of these mechanisms involve direct contact between organisms, but others result from changes in the environment caused by the antagonist. Where pathogens are involved, the environment can, of course, include the host plant itself.

Mechanisms involving direct contact between micro-organisms appear to be rather rare and until the last few years relatively few instances of hyperparasitism had been recorded. Following more detailed surveys, additional examples of direct parasitism of one micro-organism on another have now been discovered. One of these has even been adopted in a practical

Table 10.8   Mechanisms of microbial antagonism.

A. Mechanisms involving direct contact
Hyperparasitism
Mechanical obstruction
Predation
B. Mechanisms involving the environment
All environments
Competition for nutrients
Alterations in substrate pH
Production of antibiotics and other inhibitors
The host environment
Induction of phytoalexins
Immunization

scheme to control disease (see p. 211), and there may be more exciting possibilities here than have hitherto been recognized.

Many more interactions have been described where the antagonistic micro-organism affects the pathogen via the environment. Competition for nutrients may simply involve a battle between the two competing organisms for the limited supplies available in the environment, but a more subtle variant of this situation has been discovered in studies of the phylloplane. When dormant *Botrytis* spores are placed in water, some of their endogenous store of nutrients leaks out during the process of hydration. If the water droplet is sterile, these nutrients are re-absorbed as germination commences. If, however, there are bacteria in the droplet then these organisms can rapidly scavenge the nutrients before the fungus is able to regain them, and this has been shown to lead to inhibition of spore germination.

Detailed investigation of the mechanism by which *Peniophora* affects *Heterobasidion* has shown that interactions between individual hyphae are involved. In this form of antagonism, which was first discovered in studies of dung fungi, the hyphae of the antagonist grow into close contact with the victim, whose hyphae then cease to elongate and eventually die, probably due to extracellular toxins released by the antagonist. Similar interactions also occur, albeit rather rarely, between *Septoria nodorum* and some of the non-pathogenic fungi which live on the surfaces of barley leaves.

Future developments in biological control

Biological control encompasses a wide variety of approaches to the problem of restricting disease development. A comprehensive account of all these methods has been given by Baker & Cook. They describe how in many instances beneficial techniques have been practised for decades but the underlying mechanisms of control have only recently been recognized. In other cases, biological control involves alterations to established agricultural routines with the specific aim of limiting disease.

Despite recent advances, it is likely that we have scarcely begun to appreciate the extent to which biological control operates in field conditions. Indeed, in our ignorance we have undoubtedly sometimes adopted agricultural practices which actually negate natural constraints on pathogens. It is obvious that this state of affairs should not continue. However, until we understand the way in which ecological factors interact to restrict disease it is unlikely that we will be able to enhance naturally occurring systems of biological control and still less initiate successful man-made control schemes.

INTEGRATED PATHOGEN/PEST MANAGEMENT

Integrated pathogen/pest management (IPM) involves the creation of systems which utilize all available methods in as compatible a manner as possible, so as to maintain the pathogen population at a level below that which would cause economic loss. IPM might thus appear to be a complex and daunting concept, but it should not be regarded as such. There is no magic formula at work, nor is the system controlled by a black box. Rather it is based on a practical, common-sense, holistic approach whereby all available information is pooled and used rationally to devise a control scheme in which none of the resources is misused, wasted or unduly emphasized.

As with biological control, much of the early progress in this approach to pathology was made by entomologists. In the late 1950s a number of problems arose in the use of insecticides. Two of these were the development of resistance to insecticides, which was correlated with the occurrence of unusually severe outbreaks of some pests, and a growing awareness of the extent of the environmental hazards associated with their use. DDT was one of the most successful insecticides at this time but its widespread use led to the emergence of resistant strains of houseflies and mosquitoes and there were also unprecedented outbreaks of spider mites and scale insects following DDT treatment. In addition, Rachael Carson in her book *Silent Spring* marshalled a strong case against the use of this compound on environmental grounds. The occurrence of such problems made it clear that attempts to combat a pest by a single strategy are doomed to failure from the start. As a result, more comprehensive, integrated systems of pest control have been developed.

Effective integrated management demands that the crop and its environs be considered as an ecosystem. It requires realistic assessments of the economic significance of disease. The ecological, sociological and financial aspects of the available control measures must be estimated. All these factors are then considered together to obtain the best possible solution or compromise to overcome the problem posed by the disease.

In the field of pest research the development of integrated management has had the practical advantage of reducing insecticide use, in some instances by as much as 50%. However, despite successes like these, microbial plant pathologists have not yet begun to take the same degree of interest in this approach to disease control. Indeed, although some schemes have been instituted for particular pathogens, this concept is still not adequately discussed in treatises on plant pathology.

There is no doubt that one of the reasons for this state of affairs is that many of the traditional control measures used against microbial plant pathogens are highly effective. In addition, it may be argued that there has always been an element of integrated control in microbial plant pathology. The planting of resistant cultivars has often been carried out in conjunction with chemical control measures, crop sanitation and rotations with different crops. Such practices were, and in some cases still are, largely empirical in origin.

Attempts are, however, being made to rationalize this situation. For example it has been demonstrated that polygenic resistance to potato late blight can mean a reduction in fungicide use of about 0.5 kg/hectare/week against that needed for cultivars possessing no resistance. Further improvements in fungicide efficiency may be obtained if the timing of sprays is governed by a forecasting system such as Blitecast (see p. 90). Consequent reductions in the number of spray applications (Table 10.9) not only result in financial economies but also reduce the mechanical damage to the crop and the levels of fungicide residues in the produce.

Table 10.9 Control of late blight of potato in small field plots sprayed with a fungicide at either weekly intervals or according to a disease forecasting system (data from Fry & Thurston, 1980).

Year	Criterion for spray application	No. of fungicide applications	Final amount of foliar blight
1973	7-day intervals	10	0.3
	Blitecast forecast	6	0.2
1974	7-day intervals	9	<0.1
	Blitecast forecast	5	<0.1
	Unsprayed	0	89.0

Footnote: In both years differences between the final amount of blight with weekly and Blitecast spray regimes were not significantly different.

Cucumber powdery mildew, *Sphaerotheca fuliginea* (Fig. 10.6), severely affects production if it becomes rampant in greenhouses. Attempts to control the pathogen using systemic fungicides were highly effective, but only for a short time (see p. 190), and there are limits to the extent to which the environment can be manipulated so as to discourage the development of the pathogen. A recent suggestion, which is currently being assessed, involves a hyperparasite of *Sphaerotheca* which has the additional advantage of being tolerant of some of the fungicides presently used against the powdery mildew. Suspensions of hyperparasite spores are applied as a spray treatment and the environment is then adjusted to favour its rapid development. The environment is subsequently kept relatively cool and humid so as to discourage the growth of the powdery mildew fungus. Fungicides are used only if the disease shows signs of becoming significant and then the formulations and application rates are tailored to cause minimum damage to the population of the hyperparasite.

In other instances, the focus is on the crop and its several diseases rather than on one disease in isolation. A good deal of success has been achieved in this respect with the sugar beet crop. This plant can be ravaged by numerous pests and diseases, and intensive research has shown how many of

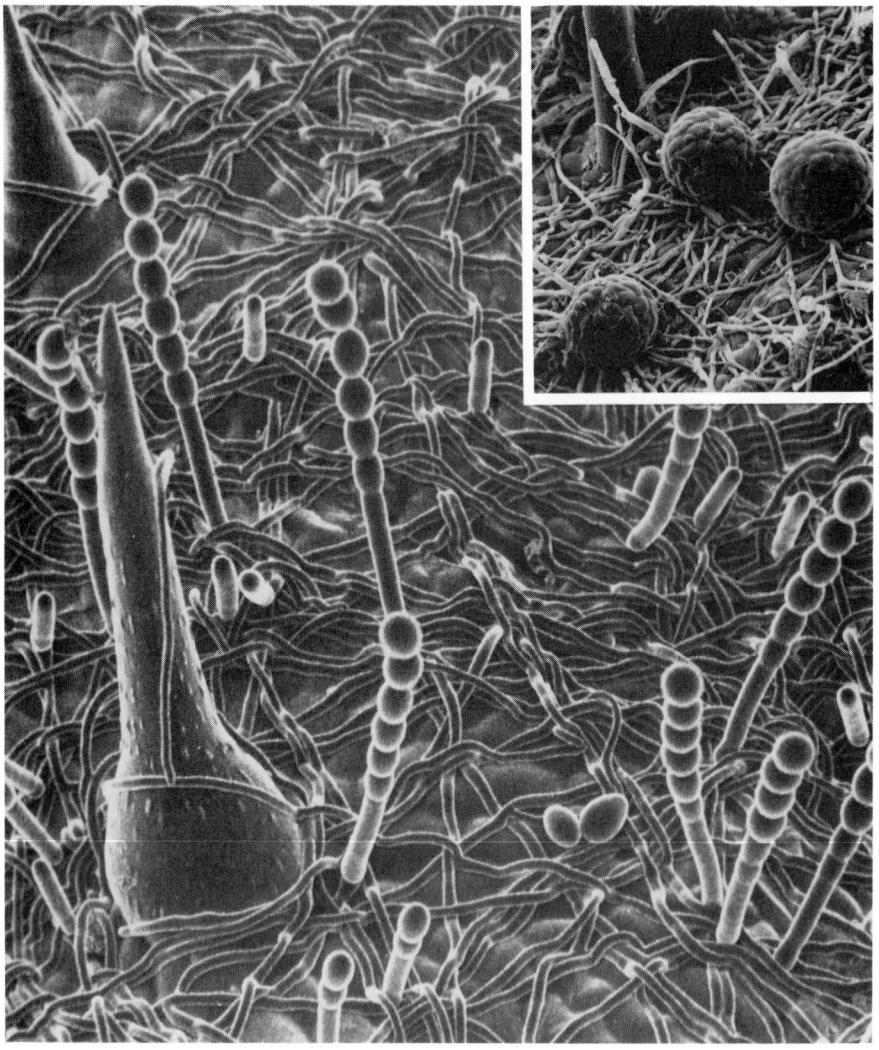

Figure 10.6 Cucumber powdery mildew (× 325) showing the superficial vegetative hyphae and the upright conidiophores, upon which are developing the chains of ovoid conidia (photograph by courtesy of ICI Plant Protection Division). Inset picture shows the developing perithecia of a powdery mildew pathogen—these structures mature and release ascospores after overwintering.

these may be controlled by one or more cultivation practices (Table 10.10). These practices are now dovetailed together to ensure that yields are maintained at a consistently high level with only a minimum outlay.

More sophisticated management of our control resources requires a realistic appraisal of disease control, as outlined above. In view of the ever-increasing demands for more food it is hard to escape the conclusion that integrated control is destined to become a vital part of our agricultural strategy. It must, however, be realized that this does not mean that chemical

Table 10.10 Integrated control measures employed to maintain high yields of sugar beet (data from Hull, 1974).

Control Measure	Disease Affected
Crop hygiene	Aphids → yellows viruses
	Aphids → mosaic virus
	Downy mildew
	Powdery mildew
	Rust
Crop rotation	Cyst nematode
	Pygmy beetle
Sowing date	Aphids → viruses
	Downy mildew
Plant spacing and cover crops	Aphids → viruses
	Ramularia leaf spot
	Curly top virus
Cultivar	Downy mildew
Pesticides	Aphids → viruses
Predators and parasites	Aphids → viruses

control is going to be phased out in the near future. Indeed in many developing countries there will be an increased use of pesticides and even in intensive agricultural systems they will remain one of the vital weapons in our war on pathogens, although their use will, one hopes, become more rational and effective.

FURTHER READING

General texts

BAKER K.F. & COOK R.J. (1974) *Biological Control of Plant Pathogens.* W.H. Freeman, San Francisco.
When this book first appeared it was hailed as an outstanding contribution to biological control theory and practice. It still provides a valuable compendium of ideas and references.

CARSON R. (1962) *Silent Spring.* Penguin, London.
The seminal book in the debate concerning the environmental impact of pesticides.

FLETCHER W.W. (1974) *The Pest War.* Basil Blackwell, Oxford.
An entertaining account of the whole field of pesticide development, with many illuminating asides which make the whole book eminently readable.

JENKYN J.F. & PLUMB R.T. eds (1981) *Strategies for the Control of Cereal Disease.* Blackwell Scientific Publications, Oxford.
Several useful chapters, especially on the philosophy of cereal breeding and the use of fungicides.

MARSH R.W. ed. (1977) *Systemic Fungicides.* Longman, London.
The second edition of this book has been expanded to include much of the rapidly increasing literature on this exciting class of pesticides.

RUSSELL G.E. (1978) *Plant Breeding for Pest and Disease Resistance.* Butterworths, London.
An exhaustive volume with full details of the breeding strategies used to create novel cultivars containing appropriate levels of disease resistance.

VAN DEN BOSCH R. & MESSENGER P.S. (1973) *Biological Control.* Intertext, New York.
This book chronicles the considerable achievements to date in introducing biological control for management of pests and weeds.

Reviews and original articles

BLAKEMAN J.P. & BRODIE I.D.S. (1976) Inhibition of pathogens by epiphytic bacteria on aerial plant surfaces. In *Microbiology of Aerial Plant Surfaces* (eds Dickinson C.H. & Preece T.F.), pp. 529–557. Academic Press, London.

BRETTELL R.I.S. & INGRAM D.S. (1979) Tissue culture in the production of novel disease-resistant plants. *Biological Reviews* **54**, 329–345.

COCKING E.C., DAVEY M.R., PENTAL D. & POWER J.B. (1981) Aspects of plant genetic manipulation. *Nature* (London) **293**, 265–270.

COMMITTEE ON CHEMICAL CONTROL, INTERNATIONAL SOCIETY OF PLANT PATHOLOGY (1981) Problems and prospects of chemical control of plant diseases. *Plant Protection Bulletin* **28**, 92–106.

CREMLYN R.J. (1977) The mode of biochemical action of some well-known fungicides. In *Herbicides and Fungicides* (ed. McFarlane N.R.), pp. 22–34. Special Publication No. 29. The Chemical Society, London.

DEKKER J. (1976) Acquired resistance to fungicides. *Annual Review of Phytopathology* **14**, 405–428.

FRY W.E. & THURSTON H.D. (1980) The relationship of plant pathology to integrated pest management. *BioScience* **30**, 665–669.

HASKELL P.T. (1977) Integrated pest control and small farmer crop protection in developing countries. *Outlook on Agriculture* **9**, 121–6.

JOHNSON R. (1981) Durable resistance: definition of, genetic control, and attainment in plant breeding. *Phytopathology* **71**, 567–8.

KRANTZ J. (1981) Hyperparasitism of biotrophic fungi. In *Microbial Ecology of the Phylloplane* (ed. Blakeman J.P.), pp. 327–352. Academic Press, London.

MOORE L.W. (1979) Practical use and success of *Agrobacterium radiobacter* strain 84 for crown gall control. In *Soil-borne Plant Pathogens* (eds Schippers B. & Gams W.), pp. 553–568. Academic Press, London.

NELSON R.R. (1978) Genetics of horizontal resistance. *Annual Review of Phytopathology* **16**, 359–378.

ORGANISATION FOR ECONOMIC CO-OPERATION AND DEVELOPMENT (1980) The fertilizers and pesticides industry. Sector Report.

WAY M.J. (1977) Integrated control—practical realities. *Outlook on Agriculture* **9**, 127–135.

Appendix
Annotated list of pathogens and the diseases they cause

Main diseases considered in the text. These are arranged according to the type of pathogen and within each group on an alphabetic basis. The letters in the notes for certain entries refer to texts in the Recommended Reading (see p. 222).

PATHOGEN	HOST	NOTES
Viruses		
Barley yellow dwarf virus	Barley, oats, wheat and over 100 other Gramineae	Persistent aphid vector controlled by aphicidal sprays applied shortly after arrival of viruliferous aphids. A, C, E, F
Bean common mosaic virus	*Phaseolus* and *Vicia* beans	Aphid vectors, control difficult. F, J
Beet mild yellowing virus	Sugar beet and other Chenopodiaceae	Vectors are *Myzus persicae* and *Aphis fabae*, control involves warning schemes plus use of insecticides, hygiene and breeding for resistance. C, E, F, J
Cacao swollen shoot virus (numerous strains or separate viruses)	Cocoa and baobab trees, mainly in West Africa	Scale-insect vectors, control by insecticides, eradicating infected trees, and resistant cultivars. C, E, F, J
Cucumber mosaic virus	Cucumber plus banana, celery, lettuce, potato, spinach, tobacco, tomato and many other plants	Non-persistent aphid vectors, rarely seed-borne, control based on aphid vector, resistance may be used in future. C, F, J, K
Grapevine fanleaf virus	Grapevine	Transmitted by persistent nematode vectors and vegetative propagation, control by cloning virus-free stocks. C, F
Grapevine leafroll virus	Grapevine	Transmitted by vegetative propagation but natural mode unknown, affects quality of wine.
Lettuce big vein virus	Lettuce and other Compositae	Transmitted by *Olpidium*, control by soil treatment to eliminate fungus e.g. steaming or chloropicrin fumigation. F
Potato leafroll virus	Potato plus tomato and other Solanaceae	Persistent aphid vectors, control by heat treatment of tubers to give virus-free plants, breeding may become important. C, E, F
Potato mop-top virus	Potato and other Solanaceae	Transmitted by the powdery scab fungus, *Spongospora subterranea*, control difficult. C, F

PATHOGEN	HOST	NOTES
Potato virus X	Potato and other Solanaceae	Mechanically transmitted, also transmitted by wart pathogen *Synchytrium endobioticum*, resistant cultivars available or use virus-free seed. C, E, F
Raspberry ringspot virus	Raspberry, tomato, gooseberry and other plants	Nematode and seed transmitted, control involves killing nematodes. C, F
Tobacco mosaic virus	Tobacco, tomato and many other plants	Mechanically transmitted, also on and in seeds, control in tomato by prior inoculation with avirulent strains of the virus and by using resistant cultivars. A, C, E, F
Tobacco rattle virus	Tobacco plus potato, sugar beet and over 100 other species	Persistent nematode vectors, also mechanically transmitted, causes spraing browning arcs in tubers, common on light soils, control by chemical treatments to kill nematodes, or resistant cultivars. C, F
Tulip-breaking virus	Tulip	Mechanically transmitted. F

Viroid

Potato spindle tuber viroid	Potato and tomato	Spread by handling tubers, also in seed and insects, control by planting viroid-free stock. A, F

Mycoplasmas

Apple rubbery wood	Apple	Transmitted by budding or grafting, control by heating affected tissues. F
Aster yellows	Carrot, celery, lettuce, onion and many ornamentals	Leafhopper vector, control by removing weed hosts or use insecticides. A
Citrus stubborn	Oranges, grapefruit	Spread by vegetative propagation and probably by leafhoppers, use disease-free stock, sanitation and antibiotics which give remission of symptoms for a useful period. A
Coconut lethal yellowing	Coconut and other palms	Vector not known, control by sanitation, resistant trees and tetracycline antibiotics. A
Corn stunt	Maize	Leafhopper vectors, control by planting resistant cultivars. A

Bacteria

Agrobacterium tumefaciens	Apple, raspberry, rose, sweet pea, blackberry and many other plants	Crown gall disease, does not always have drastic effect on growth, difficult to isolate organism from galls, which can be induced by migratory cells (e.g. in blackberry), control now using antagonist (see Chapter 10). A, K
Corynebacterium insidiosum	Alfalfa	Wilt, enters through wounds, seed-borne, on debris in soil, control by resistant cultivars, short rotations, avoid wounding plants or transferring pathogen to new areas. A

216

PATHOGEN	HOST	NOTES
Erwinia amylovora	Apple, pear, quince, hawthorn and other Rosaceae	Fireblight, control by pruning and well-timed sprays depending upon weather, especially when temperature in excess of 16°C, varieties differ markedly in susceptibility, use copper and streptomycin bactericoides. A, E
Erwinia carotovora (vars *carotovora* and *atroseptica*)	Potato	Soft rot of tubers and black leg of haulm, control by maintaining low incidence in seed crops by inspection and rogueing, keep produce dry. A, J
Erwinia tracheiphila	Cucumber and other cucurbits	Bacterial wilt of cucurbits. A
Pseudomonas citri	Citrus	Citrus canker.
Pseudomonas glycinea (pathovar of *Ps. syringae*)	Soybeans	Bacterial blight. A
Pseudomonas phaseolicola (pathovar of *Ps. syringae*)	*Phaseolus* beans	Halo blight, control by planting pathogen-free, certified seed (see Chapter 6). A
Pseudomonas solanacearum	Potato plus banana, eggplant, groundnut, tobacco and tomato	Wilt diseases including Moko disease of banana, rotations with other crops, plant resistant cultivars and avoid mechanical transmission. A, K
Pseudomonas tabaci (pathovar of *Ps. syringae*)	Tobacco	Wildfire, control using resistant cultivars, seed disinfection, seedbed sterilization and sprays of streptomycin. A, K
Streptomyces scabies	Potato	Common scab on tubers, favoured by low soil moisture during tuber development and by high pH. J

Fungi

Albugo candida	Crucifers	White blister rust. J, K
Alternaria alternata	Cotton and many other plants	Leaf spots and blights, not easily controlled by fungicides, use resistant cultivars. A
Alternaria kikuchiana	Japanese pear	Black-spot disease.
Alternaria solani	Potato, tomato	Early blight of foliage, common in warmer countries. K
Armillaria mellea	Conifers, including pine, spruce and cedar, and broad-leaved trees	Butt-rot (heart wood decayed) or general necrosis, control by removing diseased tissue which acts as food base, fungicides. A, B, K
Botrytis cinerea	Herbaceous plants, especially lettuce, tomato and other protected crops	Grey mould on juvenile and senescing tissues, control by fungicides (dicarboximides, dichlofluanid and benzimidazoles), but fungicide resistance becoming widespread. A, J, K
Botrytis fabae	*Phaseolus* beans	Chocolate spot, probably seed-borne, control using benzimidazoles. K
Bremia lactucae	Lettuce and other composites	Downy mildew, many races known, control by reducing humidity and by fungicides (acylalanine/dithiocarbamate mixtures). J
Ceratocystis fagacearum	Oak	Wilt disease, spreads by root grafts and beetle vectors, control difficult, disease contained rather than eliminated. A, K

PATHOGEN	HOST	NOTES
Ceratocystis fimbriata	Sweet potato	Black rot.
Ceratocystis ulmi	Elm	Dutch elm disease, bark beetle vectors, benzimidazole fungicides injected under pressure into trees. A
Claviceps purpurea	Rye, wheat, barley, oats and many grasses	Ergot, control by using pathogen-free seed. J
Colletotrichum circinans	Onion	Smudge disease. A
Colletotrichum lagenarium	Cucurbits including watermelon, cantaloupe and cucumber	Anthracnose, use disease-free seed, fungicides, resistant cultivars and long rotations. A
Colletotrichum lindemuthianum	*Phaseolus* beans	Anthracnose, control by using certified, pathogen-free seed. K
Cronartium ribicola	White pine/currant and gooseberry	Blister rust, eradicate alternate hosts with herbicides, prune out infected branches and use resistant trees. A
Diplocarpon rosae	Rose	Black spot on foliage, remove infected debris, spray with benzimidazole, dodemorph or captan. A
Dothidella ulei	Rubber	Leaf spot, endemic in South America but not in Malaysia, from which it is excluded by quarantine.
Epichloe typhina	Cocksfoot and other grasses	Choke disease, no control measures available. J
Erysiphe graminis	Wheat, barley, oats and many grasses	Powdery mildew, control by breeding and systemic fungicides, such as tridemorph and ethirimol. E, J, K
Fomes lignosus	Rubber	White root disease, pentachloronitrobenzene used to arrest growth of rhizomorphs on roots. B
Fulvia (Cladosporium) fulva	Tomato	Leaf mould disease, mainly controlled by use of resistant cultivars, also sprays of benzimidazoles or dichlofluanid. E, K
Fusarium oxysporum		
f.sp. *conglutinans*	Cabbage	Cabbage yellows (a type of wilt).
f.sp. *cubense*	Banana	Panama disease, control by growing resistant varieties.
f.sp. *lycopersici*	Tomato	Wilt, control by steam sterilization resistant rootstocks, isolated systems for growing plants e.g. peat bags. A, E, K
Fusarium solani f.sp. *pisi*	Pea	Foot rot. K
Fusiccocum amygdali	Peach	Canker
Gaeumannomyces (Ophiobolus) graminis	Cereals, including wheat and barley, and grasses	Take-all or whiteheads, control by rotation to grasses or by continuous cultivation when take-all decline limits disease losses. B, J, K
Gibberella fujikuroi	Rice	Foolish seedling, Fool's rice or Bakanae disease, control by treating seed with mercury and rotating with non-susceptible crops.
Helminthosporium maydis (Cochliobolus heterostrophus)	Maize	Southern corn leaf blight, control by using resistant varieties. E, K

PATHOGEN	HOST	NOTES
Helminthosporium oryzae (*Cochliobolus miyabeanus*)	Rice	Seedling blight and leaf spot.
Helminthosporium sacchari	Sugar cane	Eyespot.
Helminthosporium (*Cochliobolus*) *victoriae*	Oats and grasses	Victoria blight, seed-borne, treat with fungicide, and also soil-borne, control difficult. E, J
Hemileia vastatrix	Coffee	Leaf rust, grow resistant varieties, spray with fungicides. A, E, K
Heterobasidion annosum (*Fomes annosus*)	Pine and other conifers	Root- and butt-rot, control using antagonistic fungus. A, B
Melampsora lini	Flax	Rust
Microsphaera alphitoides	Oak	Powdery mildew. G, K
Monilinia (*Sclerotinia*) *fructicola*	Apple, plum, and other pome fruits	Brown rot of fruit, control with benzimidazole sprays—resistance not yet reported. A
Mycosphaerella musicola	Banana	Leaf spot or Sigatoka disease, see Chapter 6, control by quarantine, sanitation and frequent fungicidal sprays. A, K
Nectria galligena	Apple, pear and many other hardwood trees	Canker disease, sanitation important with these long-lived hosts, fungicidal sprays immediately after leaf fall or use antagonistic bacteria. A, K
Olpidium brassicae	Lettuce and other plants	Root infection—mainly of interest because of its ability to transmit virus.
Penicillium digitatum	Citrus	Green mould, post-harvest rot, control by careful handling and fungicide dips to prevent spread in boxes. K
Penicillium expansum	Apple, pear	Blue mould of apple, a brown, post-harvest rot, control by benzimidazole dip.
Penicillium italicum	Citrus	Blue mould—as for green mould above, benzimidazole resistance common in both species but this compound plus diphenyl is still used to protect fruit in transit and storage. A, K
Periconia circinata	Sorghum	Milo disease, soil-borne pathogen, toxin produced (see Chapter 8). E
Peronospora farinosa	Sugar beet and other cultivated beets	Downy mildew, fungicides not used, resistant cultivars planted. E, K
Peronospora parasitica	Cabbage and many other crucifers	Downy mildew, control using acylalanine/dithiocarbamate fungicides. J
Peronospora tabacina (*P. nicotianae*)	Tobacco	Blue mould. K
Phymatotrichum omnivorum	Cotton plus alfalfa, shrubs and weeds	Texas or cotton root rot, sclerotia survive in soil, control by deep cultivation to bury sclerotia or by long rotations. A, B, K
Phytophthora erythroseptica	Potato	Pink rot of tubers. J
Phytophthora infestans	Potato	Late blight of haulm and tubers, control by spraying according to forecasts, and resistant varieties. A, E, J, K
Phytophthora megasperma	Beet, carrot, potato, spinach and crucifers	Root rot. A

PATHOGEN	HOST	NOTES
Plasmodiophora brassicae	Cabbage, turnip and other crucifers	Club root or finger and toe disease, control using calomel at transplanting and by liming soil, resistance in swedes, benzimidazoles useful on transplanted crop. A, J, K
Plasmopora viticola	Vine	Downy mildew, American grapes show resistance, fungicides also commonly used. A
Pseudoperonospora cubensis	Cucurbits	Downy mildew. A
Pseudoperonospora humuli	Hop	Downy mildew, control by sprays of acylalanine/copper mixtures. K
Pseudocerosporella herpotrichoides	Wheat, barley and grasses	Eyespot, controlled by rotation, benzimidazole sprays and resistant cultivars (see Chapter 10). J
Puccinia graminis	Form species on wheat, rye, oats and grasses	Black stem rust, control by removing alternate host (barberry), resistant cultivars or fungicides. A, E, J
Puccinia horiana	Chrysanthemum	White rust, exclusion and eradication policy in UK maintains stock free of this pathogen.
Puccinia striiformis	Wheat, barley, rye and numerous grasses	Yellow stripe rust, control by fungicides, and by planting resistant cultivars. E, J
Pyrenophora avenae	Oats	Seedling blight and leaf stripe, encouraged by cold, wet conditions, seed-borne, control by seed treatment with fungicide. J
Pythium ultimum (and other species)	Seedlings of many plants	Damping-off diseases, control by keeping soil dry and cool, incorporating fungicide in composts or sterilizing soil. A
Rhizoctonia (Corticium) solani	Seedlings of many plants *Individual hyphae juvenile & senosced tissues*	Damping-off, control use pentachloro-nitrobenzene or steam to sterilize soil. K
	Potato	Black scurf (sclerotia) on tubers and necrosis of shoots. J
	Sugar beet	Black-leg or black-root. J
Rhizopus stolonifer	Many fruits, including apple, peach, and tomatoes and storage tissues, such as sweet potatoes and peanuts	Post-harvest rots, control by careful handling, fungicidal dips and refrigeration. A, K
Rhynchosporium secalis	Barley, rye and some grasses	Leaf blotch or scald, control using resistant cultivars or benzimidazole sprays. J
Sclerotinia—see *Monilinia*		
Septoria nodorum	Wheat, barley, rye and grasses	Glume blotch, control by treatment with fungicides at G.S.59, resistant cultivars and sow early to avoid worst effects. J
Sphaerotheca fuliginea	Cucurbits	Powdery mildew, control with systemic fungicides, by manipulating the environmental conditions, and hyper-parasites. G

PATHOGEN	HOST	NOTES
Synchytrium endobioticum	Potato	Wart disease, particularly effects tubers, uncommon in UK, outbreaks of the disease must be reported and only immune varieties may then be grown. J
Taphrina deformans	Peach, almond	Peach leaf curl, control by copper or sulphur sprays at bud burst. A
Uromyces phaseoli	*Phaseolus* beans	Rust, fungicides available.
Ustilago maydis	Maize	Corn smut, control by growing resistant varieties. A
Ustilago nuda	Barley, wheat	Loose smut, control by treating seed with fungicides, such as mercury compounds or oxathiin. A, J
Venturia inaequalis	Apple	Scab, control by spraying with captan, triforine or benzimidazole compounds or use urea to promote litter decomposition and hence reduce overwintering inoculum. A, K
Verticillium albo-atrum	Hop, lucerne, potato, sugar beet, tomato	*Verticillium* wilt, strains of this pathogen are usually more virulent on one of the hosts listed, control measures vary—tomato wilt is controlled by benzimidazole drenches and resistant cultivars, hop wilt by legislation, lucerne wilt by seed treatment. J
Verticillium fungicola	Cultivated mushroom	Dry bubble disease, control with fungicides but resistant strains have become troublesome.

Recommended reading

General texts

A AGRIOS G.N. (1978) *Plant Pathology*, 2nd Ed. Academic Press, New York and London.
B GARRETT S.D. (1970) *Pathogenic Root-Infecting Fungi*. Cambridge University Press, Cambridge.
C GIBBS A. & HARRISON B. (1976) *Plant Virology: the Principles*. Edward Arnold, London.
D HEITEFUSS R. & WILLIAMS P.H. eds (1976) *Encyclopedia of Plant Physiology*, Vol. IV, *Physiological Plant Pathology*. Springer Verlag, Berlin.
E RUSSELL G.E. (1978) *Plant Breeding for Pest and Disease Resistance*. Butterworths, London.
F SMITH K.M. (1972) *A Textbook of Plant Virus Diseases*. Longman, London.
G SPENCER D.M. ed. (1978) *The Powdery Mildews*. Academic Press, London.
H STROBEL G.A. & MATHRE D.E. (1970) *Outlines of Plant Pathology*. van Nostrand Reinhold, New York.
I TARR S.A.J. (1972) *Principles of Plant Pathology*. Macmillan, London.
J WESTERN J.H. ed. (1971) *Diseases of Crop Plants*. Macmillan, London.
K WHEELER B.E.J. (1969) *An Introduction to Plant Disease*. John Wiley & Sons, London.

Index